THE LPN-TO-RN
BRIDGE
TRANSITIONS TO ADVANCE YOUR CAREER

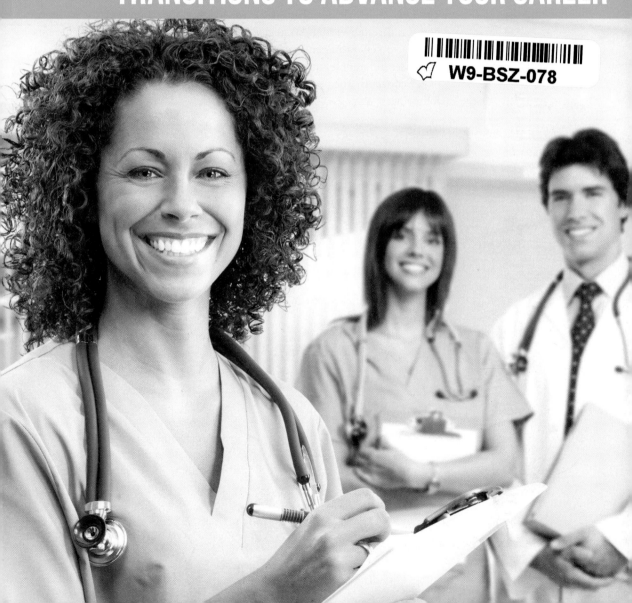

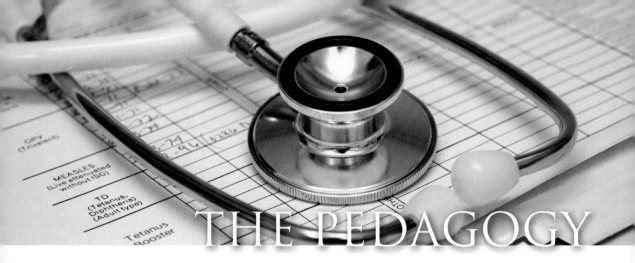

THE PEDAGOGY

The LPN-to-RN Bridge: Transitions to Advance Your Career drives comprehension through various strategies that meet the learning needs of students, while also generating enthusiasm about the topic. This interactive approach addresses different learning styles, making this the ideal text to ensure mastery of key concepts. The pedagogical aids that appear in most chapters include the following:

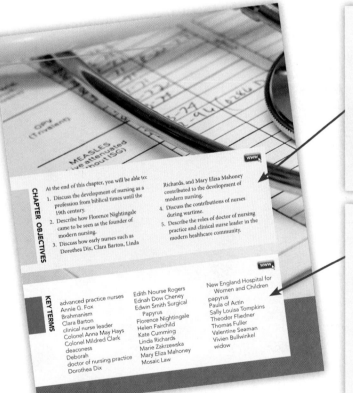

Chapter Objectives These objectives provide instructors and students with a snapshot of the key information they will encounter in each chapter. They serve as a checklist to help guide and focus study. Objectives can also be found on the companion website at **http://go.jblearning. com/terryLPN.**

Key Terms Found in a list at the beginning of each chapter, these terms will create an expanded vocabulary. The "www" icon directs students to the companion website **http:// go.jblearning.com/terryLPN** to see these terms in an interactive glossary and use flashcards and word puzzles to nail the definitions.

Scenarios Case studies encourage active learning and promote critical thinking skills in learners. Students can analyze the situation they are presented with and solve problems so they can learn how the information in the text applies to everyday practice online at **http://go.jblearning.com/terryLPN.**

6. Compare and contrast the contributions of Dorothea Dix, Clara Barton, Sally Louisa Tompkins, and Kate Cummings to nursing during the American Civil War era.
7. Compare and contrast the contributions of Linda Richards and Mary Eliza Mahoney to the development of modern nursing. Do you believe some of the same obstacles these nursing pioneers faced still exist in nursing today? Be able to support your answer.
8. Compare and contrast the contributions of Helen Fairchild and Vivien Bullwinkel to the development of modern nursing. What coping methods do you believe these heroic nurses used to help them practice nursing under such terrible conditions?

Scenarios

1. Florence Nightingale used the outbreak of the Crimean War as an opportunity to take nursing much further along the route to becoming a respectable profession. What do you believe would be needed today to progress nursing further to becoming a profession that is entered equally by both men and women?
2. Compare and contrast the requirements for a nurse in India after 1500 with those specified by Thomas Fuller, as well as those developed by Dorothea Dix. How did they change over that 300-year period of time, and how did they remain relatively unchanged?
3. Develop a set of qualifications to be a nurse in the 21st century. How do your requirements compare with those for an Indian nurse, those developed by Thomas Fuller, and those specified by Dorothea Dix?
4. Consider the hardships faced by nurses during the various wartime theaters of World War II. Do you believe today's modern nurse would be able to cope as well as these nurses did when faced with similar challenges? Be able to support your answer.
5. What preparation do you believe is needed for the modern nurse to be equipped to deal with a prison-of-war situation such as that faced by the nurses on the island of Corregidor during World War II?
6. How do you believe the role of the nurse changed from World War I to World War II? How do you believe the role of the nurse was affected by changes that occurred in modern medicine during this period of time?
7. Create a table that compares the hardships experienced, role(s) served, and circumstances under which nurses provided care in World War I, World War II, and the Vietnam War.

Critical Thinking Questions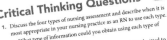

1. Discuss the four types of nursing assessment and describe when it is most appropriate in your nursing practice as an RN to use each type.
   a. What type of information could you obtain using each type of nursing assessment?
   b. You are caring for Mr. Smith, a patient who was just admitted to the medical-surgical floor complaining of persistent left upper quadrant abdominal pain. Describe how you might be required to use each of the four types of nursing assessment during your care of Mr. Smith during a 12-hour shift.
2. You are the nurse manager of a nursing unit that is attempting to be more thorough in its documentation of the daily use of the nursing process. One of the personnel that you recently hired is a new graduate licensed practical nurse who is uncertain as to how the nursing process should be used in his daily patient care. Explain in simplified terms how he should be expected to use the nursing process daily.
3. In your job as a nurse manager, you find the hospital education department has just purchased some computer software that will generate nursing diagnoses based on the input of some basic information. You overhear one of the new nurses express relief that "now we have premade diagnoses, and we don't have to figure out how they can be individualized!" Explain how you would intervene to counsel this nurse on the importance of individualizing nursing diagnoses to the specific patient.

Scenarios

1. You are caring for Mr. Jones, a 52-year-old man who drove himself to the Emergency Department and presented complaining of persistent chest pain and pressure. He smokes one pack of cigarettes daily, is morbidly obese, and reports being severely stressed at his job as an accountant. His wife is a pharmaceutical representative who travels approximately 4 days per week. Together they have two teenage boys. Mr. Smith has a 28-year-old daughter from his first marriage who is married and expecting her first baby.
   Assess this situation thoroughly and try to identify all possible nursing diagnoses. When you identify a nursing diagnosis, also identify an etiology for it as well as defining characteristics, if you believe this will strengthen the diagnosis.

Critical Thinking Questions Each chapter includes critical thinking questions that students can work on individually or in a group after reading through the material. The "www" icon directs students to the companion website **http://go.jblearning.com/terryLPN** to delve deeper into concepts by completing these exercises online.

6. Consider the patient described in scenario 4. Use the health belief model to describe the perceptions and cues to action affecting the patient as she attempts to adopt new health-promoting behaviors.
7. You have been put in charge of a task force because there is an increased public awareness of a particular genetic syndrome because there is an increased incidence of the disease in your community. Design a way to disseminate information about the disease at the individual, group, and community levels.
8. Consider the characteristics of hardiness: control, commitment, and challenge. Based on these characteristics, do you believe you possess hardiness as an individual? Why or why not? Be able to support your answer.

NCLEX® Questions

Using the information you obtained from studying this chapter, go online to complete the following NCLEX®-format review questions. Visit http://go.jblearning.com/terryLPN using the access code in the front cover of your book. This interactive resource allows you to answer each question and instantly review your results. Practice until you can answer at least 75% successfully, and then try to improve your score with each successive attempt.

Match the descriptor with the appropriate model.

1. precontemplation
2. perceived susceptibility
3. alarm reaction
4. self-efficacy
5. resistance
6. reflective self awareness
7. perceived barrier
8. preparation
9. exhaustion
10. biopsychosocial complexity
11. cues to action
12. contemplation
13. change-stability balance
14. behavioral self-regulation
15. perceived threat

NCLEX® Questions Students can prepare for the licensure exam by reviewing these questions in the book, or by going to the companion website **http://go.jblearning.com/terryLPN** where they can submit their answers and instantly review their results.

6. Your patient has an order for drug F 250 mg. The medication arrives from the hospital pharmacy as an oral suspension of 125 mg/5 ml. How many ml do you give to administer the correct dosage?
7. The physician orders your patient to receive drug G 75 mg. Your floor stocks a vial of the medication that contains 100 mg/ml. How many ml do you give to administer the correct dosage? (Round your answer to the nearest tenth.)
8. A patient has been ordered 0.25 mg of drug H. How many grams of this medication does this patient receive?
9. The patient has been ordered to receive 2 grains of a drug. The bottle is labeled 120 mg/ml. How many milliliters do you administer?
10. The physician ordered drug Q 5 mg by mouth for your patient. The medication is supplied as 2.5 mg of medication per tablet. How many tablets do you give to administer the correct dosage?

For more information on the topics in this chapter and others, please see Appendix on p. 299 for a list of web links to additional resources.

References

Burke, A. (2005). Calculation of dosages and solutions: Ratio and proportion. Retrieved from http://www.nurseceusonline.com/viewcourse/20-67010-p .htm
Cornett, E., & Blume, D. (1991). Dosages and solutions: A programmed approach to meds and math. Philadelphia, PA: F.A. Davis.
Curren, A. (2008). Math for Meds: Dosages and solutions. Florence, KY: Delmar.
Diehl, L. (2010). Brush up on your drug calculation skills. Retrieved from http://www.nursesaregreat.com
Edmunds, M. (2006). Introduction to clinical pharmacology. St. Louis, MO: Elsevier.

For a full suite of assignments and additional learning activities, use the access code located in the front of your book to visit this exclusive website: http://go.jblearning.com/terryLPN. If you do not have an access code, you can obtain one at the site.

Web Links Links to supplemental material are included at the end of each chapter for students interested in exploring topics of interest in greater depth. Students can link directly to additional websites online at **http://go.jblearning.com/terryLPN.**

THE LPN-TO-RN BRIDGE
BRIDGE
TRANSITIONS TO ADVANCE YOUR CAREER

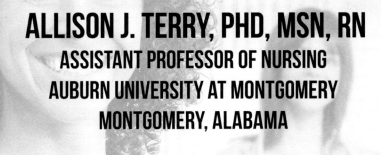

ALLISON J. TERRY, PHD, MSN, RN
ASSISTANT PROFESSOR OF NURSING
AUBURN UNIVERSITY AT MONTGOMERY
MONTGOMERY, ALABAMA

JONES & BARTLETT
LEARNING

College of the Ouachitas

World Headquarters
Jones & Bartlett Learning
5 Wall Street
Burlington, MA 01803
978-443-5000
info@jblearning.com
www.jblearning.com

Jones & Bartlett Learning books and products are available through most bookstores and online booksellers. To contact Jones & Bartlett Learning directly, call 800-832-0034, fax 978-443-8000, or visit our website, www.jblearning.com.

Substantial discounts on bulk quantities of Jones & Bartlett Learning publications are available to corporations, professional associations, and other qualified organizations. For details and specific discount information, contact the special sales department at Jones & Bartlett Learning via the above contact information or send an email to specialsales@jblearning.com.

The LPN-to-RN Bridge: Transitions to Advance Your Career is an independent publication and has not been authorized, sponsored, or otherwise approved by the owners of the trademarks or service marks referenced in this product.

Some images in this book feature models. These models do not necessarily endorse, represent, or participate in the activities represented in the images.

The author, editor, and publisher have made every effort to provide accurate information. However, they are not responsible for errors, omissions, or for any outcomes related to the use of the contents of this book and take no responsibility for the use of the products and procedures described. Treatments and side effects described in this book may not be applicable to all people; likewise, some people may require a dose or experience a side effect that is not described herein. Drugs and medical devices are discussed that may have limited availability controlled by the Food and Drug Administration (FDA) for use only in a research study or clinical trial. Research, clinical practice, and government regulations often change the accepted standard in this field. When consideration is being given to use of any drug in the clinical setting, the health care provider or reader is responsible for determining FDA status of the drug, reading the package insert, and reviewing prescribing information for the most up-to-date recommendations on dose, precautions, and contraindications, and determining the appropriate usage for the product. This is especially important in the case of drugs that are new or seldom used.

Additional credits appear on page 320, which constitutes a continuation of the copyright page.

Production Credits

Publisher: Kevin Sullivan
Acquisitions Editor: Amanda Harvey
Editorial Assistant: Sara Bempkins
Associate Production Editor: Cindie Bryan
Marketing Manager: Elena McAnespie
Associate Marketing Manager: Katie Hennessy
V.P., Manufacturing and Inventory Control: Therese Connell

Composition: Publishers' Design and Production Services, Inc.
Cover Design: Michael O'Donnell
Rights & Photo Research Associate: Lauren Miller
Cover Image: © Kurhan/ShutterStock, Inc.
Chapter Opener Image: © Amy Walters/ShutterStock, Inc.
Printing and Binding: Courier Kendallville
Cover Printing: Courier Kendallville

To order this product, use ISBN: 978-1-4496-7450-2

Library of Congress Cataloging-in-Publication Data
Terry, Allison J.
The LPN-to-RN bridge : transitions to advance your career / Allison J. Terry. -- 1st ed.
        p. ; cm.
  Includes bibliographical references and index.
  ISBN 978-1-4496-4604-2 (pbk.) -- ISBN 1-4496-4604-2 (pbk.)
  I. Title.
  [DNLM: 1. Career Mobility. 2. Nurses. 3. Nursing Process. 4. Nursing, Practical. 5. Nursing. WY 16.1]
  610.7306'9--dc23
                              2011046527
6048

Printed in the United States of America
16 15 14 13 12   10 9 8 7 6 5 4 3 2 1

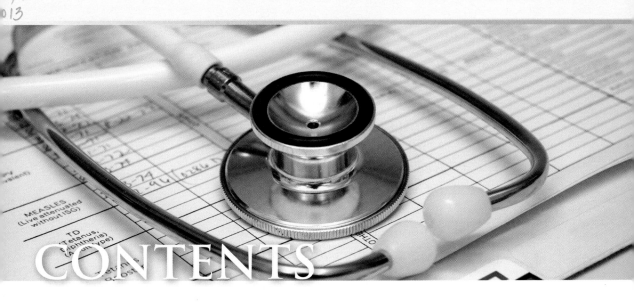

CONTENTS

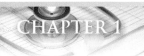

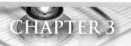

CHAPTER 3

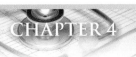

Nursing Theory   85

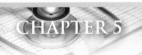

Change Process   119

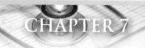

CHAPTER 7   Health Promotion   143

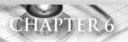

CHAPTER 6   Legal–Ethical Aspects of Nursing   167

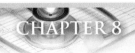

Cultural Aspects of Nursing   193

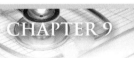

Calculation of Dosages and Solutions   221

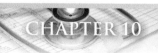

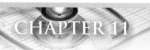

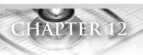

CHAPTER 12

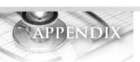

APPENDIX

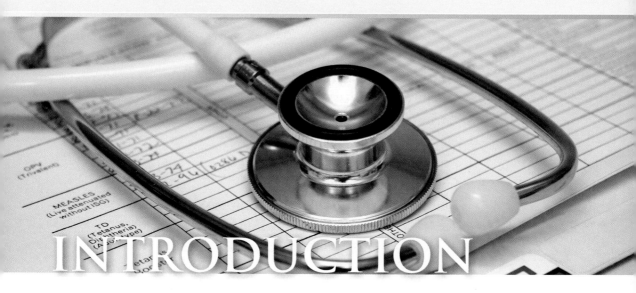

INTRODUCTION

The nursing profession is a multi-faceted one that is struggling to adapt to a healthcare environment that is changing almost moment by moment. One of the most dedicated segments of the nursing population is that of the licensed practical nurses (LPNs) who serve in a variety of clinical areas. Their professionalism is further demonstrated when they opt to continue their education by obtaining an Associate's Degree in Nursing (ADN) or a Bachelor of Science in Nursing degree (BSN). This text is designed to give these dedicated professionals the tools that they will need not only to progress further in their nursing program, but to also assume their places as nurse leaders in the healthcare community.

Because the LPN who is continuing his or her education is already highly motivated to become an even more useful contributor to the healthcare community at the local, state, national, and even global levels, it is the intent of the author to provide these nurses with a text that is both practical and user-friendly. As such, it includes information on the following areas:

- < History of nursing as a profession
- < Communication as a registered nurse
- < The nursing process
- < Nursing theory
- < Change process
- < Health promotion
- < Legal and ethical considerations
- < Cultural considerations

‹ Dosage and solutions calculations
‹ Roles of the registered nurse
‹ Evidence-based practice
‹ Clinical decision-making as a registered nurse

Because most of these nurses are practicing clinically in healthcare organizations, scenarios and critical thinking exercises are included that utilize clinical situations as well as management dilemmas that will already be familiar to them. Key terms are defined to provide additional clarity, and chapter objectives are included to assist students in designing a plan for chapter study.

A chapter on dosage and solutions calculations is included in the text in an attempt to alleviate some of the anxiety attached this topic. In addition, both ratio and proportion and dimensional analysis methods are included so that students can use the type that best fits their learning style. Multiple practice problems are included to increase the level of proficiency in this area.

In an effort to prepare these nurses to successfully complete the NCLEX® licensure examination to practice as a registered nurse (RN), NCLEX®-style review questions have also been included along with helpful web links that will supply additional information on many of topics included in the text. The accompanying website should be particularly helpful to nurses who are comfortable with electronic charting and other computerized documentation and prefer it to the standard handwritten format.

Finally, the author acknowledges the inability to generate a "one-size-fits-all" textbook that will meet the needs of every LPN who ever decides to further his or her education and become an RN. Because of the rich diversity of nurses who have chosen to devote their lives to patient care, this is unlikely to occur. Therefore, the author welcomes comments and suggestions from readers that will serve to make future editions of this text even more user-friendly and more likely to be a book that nurses will go to as a reference again and again.

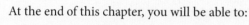

CHAPTER OBJECTIVES

At the end of this chapter, you will be able to:

1. Discuss the development of nursing as a profession from biblical times until the 19th century.
2. Describe how Florence Nightingale came to be seen as the founder of modern nursing.
3. Discuss how early nurses such as Dorothea Dix, Clara Barton, Linda Richards, and Mary Eliza Mahoney contributed to the development of modern nursing.
4. Discuss the contributions of nurses during wartime.
5. Describe the roles of doctor of nursing practice and clinical nurse leader in the modern healthcare community.

KEY TERMS

advanced practice nurses
Annie G. Fox
Brahmanism
Clara Barton
clinical nurse leader
Colonel Anna May Hays
Colonel Mildred Clark
deaconess
Deborah
doctor of nursing practice
Dorothea Dix

Edith Nourse Rogers
Ednah Dow Cheney
Edwin Smith Surgical Papyrus
Florence Nightingale
Helen Fairchild
Kate Cumming
Linda Richards
Marie Zakrzewska
Mary Eliza Mahoney
Mosaic Law

New England Hospital for Women and Children
papyrus
Paula of Actin
Sally Louisa Tompkins
Theodor Fliedner
Thomas Fuller
Valentine Seaman
Vivien Bullwinkel
widow

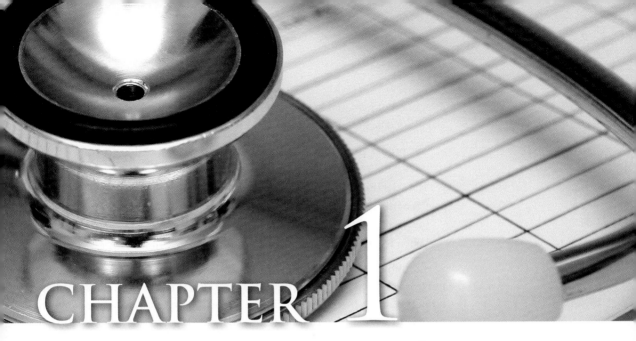

CHAPTER 1

History of Nursing as a Profession

Origins of Nursing

Nursing has been referred to as both the oldest art and the youngest profession. Its origins can be traced back to the dawn of civilization through the traditional mother–child relationship as well as to the important role of the village healer in many primitive societies. However, in more sophisticated societies such as that of ancient Egypt the importance of the nursing discipline became evident, as nurses assisted in the recovery of patients experiencing traumatic injuries, such as those sustained on the battlefield.

A *papyrus* dating back to the 17th century B.C., known as the *Edwin Smith Surgical Papyrus*, is one of the oldest documents pertaining to medicine. It is the earliest known surgical prototype textbook and lists the proper surgical treatment for a variety of traumatic injuries that begin with the head and proceed downward anatomically. Although magic was considered a major part of medical treatment at the time, the Edwin Smith papyrus only resorts to use of magic with one described case, relying instead on descriptions of logical treatment of patients (Tour Egypt, 2010).

The origins of many of the practices still used in modern nursing can be seen in the directives of the *Mosaic Law* that was followed by the ancient Israelites from the 15th century B.C. until the first century A.D. when the Jews began to be dispersed throughout the known world. As in many societies of that era, responsibility for the health of the public rested with the male-dominated priestly tribe of the Levites. The people were taught to prevent disease through a regimen of personal hygiene and specific times set aside for work, rest, and sleep. Specific and detailed instructions were provided regarding

- The proper treatment of women during pregnancy, childbirth, and menstruation
- The selection of food that met dietary requirements
- Recognizing communicable disease so priests could be notified of an outbreak
- When to implement quarantine procedures

The Bible has the distinction of being the document that records the first nurse mentioned by name in history. *Deborah* was recorded in the 24th chapter of the book of Genesis as being the nurse of Rebekah, who was traveling to meet her future husband, Isaac (Donahue, 1996).

Hygiene and the prevention of illness were further emphasized by Indian *Brahmanism* after 1500 B.C. The religion's teachings included topics such as medicine and surgery. Indian surgery was considered to be the most highly skilled of any of the known ancient civilizations.

Brahmanism, also referred to as Hinduism, further emphasized recognizing symptoms unique to specific disease processes, such as those specific to diabetes mellitus. One ancient Indian document specified the roles fulfilled by each member of a medical team, with the nurse responsible for knowledge of medication preparation in addition to "cleverness," devotion to the patient, and purity of both mind and body. Nurses are frequently referred to in Indian historical documents, although they were usually men or, in rare instances, older women. However, it is important to note that at this time in Indian history, nurses were already required to exhibit exceptional standards, skill at their craft, and a high level of integrity. Documentation from this period in India specified the characteristics required of a nurse (Donahue, 1996):

- Appropriate behavior
- Cleanliness
- Devotion to employer
- Kind
- Skilled at every type of service
- Clever in general
- Able to cook
- Skilled in bathing a patient
- Skilled in providing massage
- Able to assist a patient in walking and moving about
- Skilled in bed making

‹ Able to prepare or compound medications as needed

‹ Skilled in caring for a patient that had a difficulty recovery

‹ Always willing to carry out any act, whether commanded by the physician or the patient

In this period in history, nursing as a vocation was predominantly comprised of males. However, after the third century A.D. the gradual entrance of women into nursing was affected primarily by three factors: the improvement in the social stature of women in the Roman Empire, the teachings of Christianity regarding the equality of men and women in service to God, and the requirement of Christians to continue the work of Christ with the neglected poor. As the Christian church began to assume care of the poor and the sick of the community, women as well as men began to share this task.

Among women, *deaconesses* and *widows* began to emerge as nurses and became the prototype for the modern community health nurse. Deaconesses worked equally with male deacons and were usually required to be unmarried or widowed. Their role as visiting nurses was carried out in addition to attending to the spiritual needs of their parishioners. Widows also served as visiting nurses for the poor and were usually required to swear a vow of chastity, leading to their ultimate development into nuns. A counterpoint to deaconesses and widows were the matrons of the Roman Empire who had converted to Christianity. Their positions of authority in society and considerable wealth allowed them to have the freedom to lay the foundation for community health nursing (Donahue, 1996). *Paula of Actin*, in particular, was an extremely wealthy and learned Christian widow believed to be the first to train nurses systematically and to teach nursing as an art rather than as merely a service to the poor. However, at that time a well-trained nurse was still considered to be one who not only cared for the sick but also cooked, cleaned, and waited on any other individuals in residence at the moment who might require service (Moses, 2011).

Transition to Secular Nursing

As the Middle Ages progressed, eventually the Reformation developed and a clear-cut religious division resulted, generating both a Catholic Church and Protestantism. In England more so than in any other country in Europe monks and nuns were forced from monasteries, and hospitals and other facilities that had once been used to care for the poor and sick by religious orders were either closed or given over to other groups with less pure motives. For the first time nursing began to be less associated with religion.

To fill the void produced by the lack of nuns and other women with similar religious dedications, women from the lowest levels of society were often recruited and assigned nursing duties to replace a certain amount of a prison sentence. Hospitals became severely utilitarian, and sanitary conditions were unknown. An 18th century hospital was described as having up to six patients stretched across the width of one bed. Patients never received bed baths, and it was standard practice for a patient with a highly contagious disease to be laid in the same bed with a patient who had a reasonably treatable illness, because the cause of infection was not understood at that point in history (Donahue, 1996).

It was at this time that men seemed to take their exit from nursing. After this period, nursing in Catholic countries was carried out by women in some type of religious order, whereas in Protestant countries nursing began to be seen as a female-dominated occupation. However, leadership of hospitals was almost always a male function, and virtually no authority was given to the women who provided oversight of the nurses hired to carry out the menial chores that were then considered to be "nursing." Because of the low character of many of the women who were acting as nurses at that time, an attempt was made to develop qualifications for women who sought to function as nurses in hospitals. The set developed by *Thomas Fuller*, an English physician, was as follows (Donahue, 1996):

< Middle aged
< Healthy, particularly free from "vapors" and coughing
< Capable of being at the bedside throughout the course of the entire illness
< Ready to respond at the first call of the patient
< Capable of speaking very little, and then only in low tones, and able to walk softly
< Having keen eyes to observe any alteration in the patient's color, manner, or growth
< Able to do "everything the best way"
< Able to do everything quickly
< Clean in her habits
< Well tempered and able to humor the sick person
< Cheerful and pleasant and never cross or sad
< Capable of observing the patient both night and day
< Not subject to practicing gluttony, drinking, or smoking
< Following the physician's orders carefully
< Childless (**Table 1-1**)

Emergence of Modern Nursing

Modern nursing had its genesis in the efforts of *Theodor Fliedner*, a Lutheran minister who revived the order of deaconesses after contact with the Mora-

TABLE 1-1 Comparison of Qualifications for Nurses from 1500s–1700s

Qualifications for Nurses in India after 1500	Qualifications for Nurses Developed by Dr. Thomas Fuller
appropriate behavior	middle-aged
cleanliness	healthy, free from "vapors" and coughing
devotion to the employer	able to be at the bedside throughout the course of the entire illness
kind	cheerful, pleasant, never cross or sad
skilled at every type of service	able to do "everything the best way"
clever in general	able to do everything quickly
able to cook	capable of speaking very little, in low tones, and able to walk softly
skilled in bathing a patient	having keen eyes to observe any alteration in patient's color, manner, or growth
skilled in providing massage	clean in her habits
able to assist a patient in walking and moving about	well-tempered and able to humor the sick person
skilled in bedmaking	able to observe the patient night and day
able to prepare or compound medications as needed	not subject to gluttony, drinking, or smoking
skilled in caring for a patient that had a difficulty recovery	ready to respond at the first call of the patient
willing to carry out any act, whether directed by physician or patient	following the physician's orders carefully
	having no children

vians, who had revived the use of deaconesses in 1745. Recognizing the great need these individuals had filled in the healthcare community of the time, Pastor Fliedner founded a hospital and training center at Kaiserswerth, Germany in 1836. By 1850 the renown of the Deaconess Institute had spread beyond the borders of Germany into other European countries, and *Florence Nightingale* chose to come there for instruction at that time (Wentz, 1936).

Miss Nightingale was born in 1820 into a wealthy English family that was progressive enough to see the benefits of a thorough education for both men and women. At a time when even wealthy women received only a rudimentary education, she was schooled in various languages as well as science and mathematics. As an adult traveling in Europe she noted various facilities where

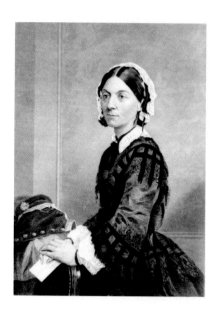

nursing was taught in systematic curriculums, thus fueling her already burning desire to attain some type of life work involving the care of others. Her parents objected to her affiliation with any hospital because of the terrible conditions that existed in these facilities at the time, with the worst such hospitals in England.

By 1854 the Crimean War had broken out, and English newspapers were filled with reports of the appalling care being provided to soldiers in English field hospitals. The care provided in French field hospitals was known to be far superior, primarily due to the efforts of the French Sisters of Charity, who had accompanied France's expedition to the Crimea in large numbers to care for the wounded. Miss Nightingale had previously become acquainted with England's Secretary of War, who was so impressed with her and her desire to work with the sick and the dying that he wrote to her asking for her help in organizing the care of the English wounded in Turkey (Donahue, 1996).

By October 1854 Miss Nightingale had been appointed superintendent over the female nurses in the English field hospitals in Turkey and sailed for Scutari along with 38 nurses. Upon her arrival she found four miles of beds holding approximately 3,500 wounded patients in a space designed for 1,700 men. The only light was given off by candles jammed into empty beer bottles, and an open sewer ran under the building. There was no water, soap, towels, knives or forks, or clothing for the patients and very little edible food. The death rate was slightly over 42%. To change the hospital from merely a storehouse for the dying into an area where the seriously ill and wounded could convalesce, Miss Nightingale opted to establish five kitchens for decent food preparation and a laundry as well as areas where recuperating soldiers could read and listen to music. In the evening she frequently made rounds alone with her lantern to observe the progress of the most critical patients, acquiring the now-famous title of "The Lady with the Lamp." Within 6 months of the implementation of the hygienic measures that Miss Nightingale insisted upon, the mortality rate in the hospital dropped to 2.2% (Donahue, 1996).

As a result of Florence Nightingale's growing fame from engineering the monumental change in English military health care and the gratitude she received from the British public, she achieved enough influence to develop a training program for nurses in a school devoted solely to this purpose. This was developed despite the objections of many English physicians who believed that such training was unnecessary because the nurse was essentially in the same position as a "housemaid" and therefore required no special training or instruction (Donahue, 1996).

Nursing During the Civil War

The development of nursing in America was a slow process, with the first nurses being servants, criminals, and paupers who cared for the sick. During the 17th and 18th centuries in America nurses from various religious orders were asked to come in and reform hospitals that had become obstacles to a patient's recovery rather than assisting with the recovery process. However, this changed with *Dorothea Dix*. Miss Dix was the superintendent of female nurses for the Union Army during the Civil War and was given the authority to organize hospitals for the care of the wounded soldiers, appoint nurses to serve in such field hospitals, and oversee the distribution of supplies for the troops. Although not a trained nurse by profession, Miss Dix had a wealth of administrative and organizational skills acquired during her efforts 20 years earlier to create more humane living conditions for the mentally ill and criminals in America's prisons. Like Thomas Fuller a century earlier, Miss Dix developed a set of requirements for women seeking to obtain an appointment as a nurse (Donahue, 1996):

< Between the ages of 35 and 50
< Healthy and free of chronic diseases
< "Matronly," "good conduct," "superior" education, and "serious" personality
< Neat, orderly, and industrious
< Able to produce at least two references to attest to the candidate's character, morality, integrity, and ability to care for the sick
< Obedience and conformity with developed rules
< Able to serve in this capacity for at least 3 months, with preference given to those able to serve for longer periods (**Tables 1-2** and **1-3**)

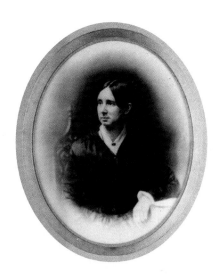

Another woman making a contribution to the war effort was *Clara Barton*, who independently organized and operated a huge war relief effort on behalf of the Union Army. She often used her own money to supply the recuperating soldiers with adequate food, clothing, bedding, and medical supplies. After the War she learned of the existence of the International Red Cross and worked with this organization for several years. She soon began efforts to organize an American Red Cross, which did not come to fruition until 1882. Miss Barton served as the first president of the American Red Cross and gave her home to be its national headquarters (Barton, 1904).

TABLE 1-2 Comparison of Qualifications for Nurses from 1700s–1800s

Qualifications for Nurses Developed by Dr. Thomas Fuller	Qualifications for Nurses Developed by Dorothea Dix
middle-aged	between the ages of 35 and 50
healthy, free from "vapors" and coughing	healthy and free of chronic diseases
able to be at the bedside throughout the course of the entire illness	able to produce at least two references regarding character, morality, integrity, and ability to care for the sick
cheerful, pleasant, never cross or sad	"serious" personality
able to do "everything the best way"	able to serve for at least three months; preference given to those able to serve longer
able to do everything quickly	superior education
capable of speaking very little, in low tones, and able to walk softly	matronly
having keen eyes to observe any alteration in patient's color, manner, or growth	neat, orderly
clean in her habits	good conduct
well-tempered and able to humor the sick person	industrious
able to observe the patient night and day	obedience and conformity with developed rules
not subject to gluttony, drinking, or smoking	
ready to respond at the first call of the patient	
following the physician's orders carefully	
having no children	

The Confederacy also saw its share of women who made significant contributions to the developing profession of nursing, with *Sally Louisa Tompkins* and *Kate Cumming* being the most famous. Sally Louisa Tompkins was born into a wealthy Virginia family and responded to the Confederate government's call for the public to assist in caring for the wounded. Miss Tompkins founded Robertson Hospital in Richmond in 1861 and subsidized it primarily with her own funds. To prevent the hospital from being taken over by the military, Miss

TABLE 1-3 Comparison of Qualifications for Nurses from 1500s–1800s

Qualifications for Nurses in India after 1500	Qualifications for Nurses Developed by Dr. Thomas Fuller	Qualifications for Nurses Developed by Dorothea Dix
appropriate behavior	middle-aged	between the ages of 35 and 50
cleanliness	healthy, no "vapors" or coughing	healthy and free of chronic diseases
devotion to the employer	able to be at bedside throughout entire illness	able to produce at least two references regarding character, morality, integrity, and ability to care for the sick
kind	cheerful, pleasant, never cross or sad	"serious" personality
skilled at every type of service	able to do "everything the best way"	able to serve for at least three months; preference given if serving longer
clever in general	able to do everything quickly	superior education
able to cook	speaking very little, in low tones, and able to walk softly	matronly
skilled in bathing a patient	keen eyes to observe any alteration in patient's color, manner, or growth	neat, orderly
skilled in providing massage	clean in her habits	good conduct
able to assist a patient in walking and moving about	well-tempered and able to humor the sick person	industrious
skilled in bedmaking	able to observe patient night and day	obedience, conformity with rules
able to prepare/compound medications as needed	not subject to gluttony, drinking, or smoking	
skilled in managing a difficult recovery	responds at the first call of the patient	
willing to carry out any act as directed by physician or patient	follows physician's orders carefully	
	having no children	

Tompkins convinced President Jefferson Davis to appoint her as captain of cavalry, making her the only woman to hold a commission in the Confederate Army. The military rank became invaluable to

> Miss Tompkins because it came with a salary that could be used to defray the costs of operating the hospital along with the privilege of accessing medical supplies and government rations. By the time the hospital closed in 1865 at the conclusion of the war, Robertson Hospital had treated a total of 1,333 patients and sustained only 73 deaths, yielding a survival rate of 94.5%. This was remarkable at a time when the radical reforms of Florence Nightingale had occurred only a decade earlier (Hagerman, 1996).

In comparison with the southern born-and-bred Sally Louisa Tompkins, Kate Cumming was originally born in Scotland but moved with her family to Mobile, Alabama, in her youth and considered herself a southerner. After joining a party of 40 women who volunteered to journey to Corinth, Mississippi, to nurse the wounded, Miss Cumming became determined to seek a permanent position in a Confederate hospital. Despite the objections of her family and the public, by 1862 she had been appointed to the position of matron, or the administrator, of the mobile field hospitals of Dr. Samuel Stout, the medical director for the Army of Tennessee. In her position of matron Miss Cumming not only managed each mobile hospital's departments and supervised its workforce but cooked, sewed, wrote letters, and foraged in the surrounding countryside for supplies. Her observations of the daily life of a confederate hospital during this time were chronicled in a diary that she kept and published after the war, giving us an invaluable picture of the hardships of that period and the strength of character of another of the great women of history who contributed to the nursing profession (Hilde, 2009).

Development of Schools of Nursing

The advent of the Civil War brought the woefully inadequate preparation of nurses in the United States to the forefront of the public's consciousness. Also, the public became more open to the idea of establishing formal training programs for nurses as more women from socially prominent families selected nursing as a vocation. The first formal instructional program for nurses is usually credited to Dr. *Valentine Seaman*, medical chief of New York Hospital. Dr. Seaman initiated a program of study for nurses in 1799 that continued until his death in 1817. This program became the framework for the entity that ultimately became Cornell University-New York Hospital School of Nursing (Engle, 1980).

As progress continued toward the development of formal training programs for nurses, the need for nurses to collaborate with female physicians in an effort to advance the professions of nursing and medicine became evident. Thus, in 1862 the *New England Hospital for Women and Children* was founded by Drs. *Marie Zakrzewska* and *Ednah Dow Cheney*. For more than 100 years it was a teaching hospital for female physicians and later nurses run by an all-female staff that offered an education comparable with that received by male physicians. It was the first facility in the Boston area to offer obstetrics, gynecology, and pediatrics in one facility (Reiskind, 1995).

The first graduate of the facility's nurses' training program was *Linda Richards* in 1873. Considered to be the first trained nurse in America, Miss Richards, whose diploma is housed in the Smithsonian Institution in Washington, DC, became the night supervisor at Bellevue Hospital and implemented major changes during her tenure: she insisted on the use of gas light at night rather than merely using a candle stub, she developed a system of charting and maintaining individual patient records, and she revealed the high mortality rate for new mothers who were dying of puerperal fever, leading to these patients being housed separately. After only 1 year Miss Richards became the superintendent of the Boston Training School, which was affiliated with Massachusetts General Hospital. Remarkably, she was able to combine administrative duties with actual bedside patient care during this time (Carnegie, 1986).

Another historically prominent figure who graduated from the nurses' training program at the New England Hospital for Women and Children was *Mary Eliza Mahoney*, the first African-American professional nurse. After working for the hospital since the age of 15, Miss Mahoney was admitted as a nursing student at the age of 33. At a time when the program admitted only one African-American student and one Jewish student into each class, she was one of only four students who completed the program out of an admitted class of 42 students. Working for many years as a private-duty nurse caring for patients in the New England area, Miss Mahoney went on to found the National Association of Colored Graduate Nurses. Today she is a member of the American Nurses Association's Nursing Hall of Fame and the National Women's Hall of Fame (Carnegie, 1986).

Nursing During World War I

Army and Navy Nurses Corp nurses who cared for casualties produced by World War I saw types of injuries that had never been produced before in wartime. The advent of both machine guns and poison gas generated horrific wounds that required new methods of treatment. The exact number of nurses who served in either Corps is uncertain because nurses tended to be grouped together into a general category of women who served in the war, but it is documented that by 1918 a total of 1,386 women were serving in the Navy Nurse Corps. The Red Cross estimates that almost 20,000 nurses were assigned to active duty during World War I and served either with the Army Nurse Corps, Navy Nurse Corps, U.S. Public Health Service, or the Red Cross overseas service. Most of these nurses served in the Army Nurse Corps (Schreiber, 1999).

Many World War I nurses worked aboard trains that could evacuate up to 400 patients from front-line facilities in an effort to move them closer to embarkation points back to the United States. Each such train, also referred to as a "moving hospital," was equipped with electric lights, steam heat, electric fans, and lavatories. However, these trains also complicated recovery, as the wounded not only contended with significant injuries but also with the jolting motion, noise, and debris associated with long-distance train travel (Schreiber, 1999).

One World War I era nurse who became famous posthumously through her poignant letters was *Helen Fairchild*. Serving as one of 64 Pennsylvania nurses who joined the American Expeditionary Force after America entered the War in 1917, Miss Fairchild wrote of standing in mud above her ankles as she assisted in the operating suite. Her chief nurse described her and her fellow nurses as working 14-hour shifts with negligible amounts of rest. Tragically, Miss Fairchild would not live to see her wonderfully descriptive letters published. While working with the British Base Hospital in France, she volunteered for front-line duty at a casualty clearing station where she was exposed to mustard gas. She was found to have a large gastric ulcer and underwent surgery to repair it, but the surgery was not successful. Miss Fairchild died in January 1918 as a result of hepatic complications from the surgery that likely were worsened as a result of her exposure to the mustard gas (Patrick, 2011).

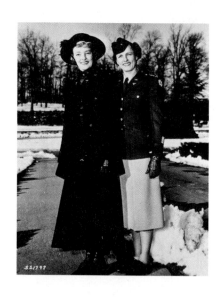

Nursing During World War II

As the prospect of war in Europe began to loom, the Army and Navy Nurse Corps had already been established and its members had served alongside the veterans of World War I. However, the federal government was slow to recognize the great need for nurses in the military until after the bombing of Pearl Harbor in December 1941. In May of that year Congresswoman *Edith Nourse Rogers* had introduced the Women's Auxiliary Army Corps bill in an effort to mobilize the much-needed nurses as well as other female personnel to assist the war effort. Concurrently, by July 1942 Congress created the WAVES (Women Accepted for Volunteer Emergency Service) through the Women's Naval Reserve Act. This group of personnel was considered from their creation to be part of the Navy rather than an auxiliary. Ultimately, more than 140,000 women served in the Women's Army Corps and at least 100,000 served as Navy WAVES (Metropolitan State College of Denver, 2004). As a result of the valiant efforts of the nurses who served in World War II, less than 4% of the American soldiers who received treatment in the field or were evacuated died either from their wounds or from disease. Reflecting the changing attitude in America toward the use of women in wartime as well as the great service being provided by the nurses in various theaters of war worldwide, by 1944 the Army was granting its nurses officers' commissions and full retirement privileges, along with pay equal to that of male counterparts and dependents' allowances. Between 1943 and 1948 the federal government provided free education to nursing students (Bellafaire, 2003).

On December 7, 1941, the day of the attack on Pearl Harbor, 82 Army nurses were stationed in Hawaii serving three Army medical facilities. Tripler Army Hospital was deluged with hundreds of casualties, and the wounded lay in the hallways awaiting their turn in the surgical suite. Medical supplies were in short supply as the wounded continued to pour into each facility, and sterile supplies ran out completely. Scissors were passed from one operating table to another, rags served double duty as both cleaning material and face masks for physicians and nurses, and operations were performed without the benefit of gloves. The chief nurse at Hickam Field, First Lieutenant *Annie G. Fox*, became the first Army nurse to receive the Purple Heart because of her example of calm, courage, and leadership during this ordeal (Bellafaire, 2003).

During most of 1941 Army nurses were increasingly sent to the Philippines as tension in that area increased. The Philippines were officially attacked by Japan on December 8, 1941, and consequently 45 nurses were sent from the island of Corregidor and Bataan to prepare two emergency hospitals. Of these hospitals, General Hospital 1 received more than 1,200 battle casualties requiring surgical procedures such as amputations within the first month. This hospital was bombed in March 1942 and received a direct hit, throwing patients from their beds. Body parts were found later that had been blown into the trees by the impact of the blast.

The dedication of the nurses serving in this area can be demonstrated by the heroism of those who stayed to care for the wounded. When it became clear that the island of Corregidor would fall, as many nurses as possible were evacuated to Australia. However, when the American forces surrendered to the Japanese on Corregidor, 55 Army nurses remained who had continued

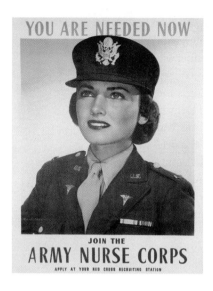

to care for the wounded at Malinta Hospital. These nurses were taken to an internment camp in Manila and remained prisoners of war until they were liberated by U.S. forces in 1945 (Doherty, 2000).

Along with starvation, tropical diseases, and deprivation of the very basic necessities of life, one group of 22 Australian nurses who had been shipwrecked in Indonesia faced being confronted and ultimately massacred by Japanese forces. The women were forced to march into the sea and then were shot as Japanese troops opened machine gun fire, despite the nurses having their Red Cross badges clearly evident. Of the 22 nurses only 1, *Vivien Bullwinkel*, received a wound that was not fatal and survived by pretending to be dead. She survived the massacre only to be captured and placed in an internment camp in Sumatra. However, in the internment camp Miss Bullwinkel was reunited with some of her nurse colleagues who had survived their shipwreck, and together they formed a support system that led to all except eight nurses surviving the camp internment (Doherty, 2000).

Nursing During the Vietnam War

The Army Nurse Corps began its service in Vietnam in 1956 when three Army nurses arrived in Saigon to teach South Vietnamese nurses nursing procedures and nursing care techniques. This number of personnel expanded until by December 1968, 900 nurses were serving in 23 Army hospitals and a convalescent center housing a combined total of more than 5,000 beds. The Army nurses in Vietnam were led by *Colonel Mildred Clark* and *Colonel Anna May Hays*, with Colonel Hays promoted to Brigadier General in 1970. Colonel Hays became the first nurse in American military history to attain general officer rank.

The nurses serving in Vietnam were on average 23 to 24 years old and were essentially new to nursing, with only 35% having more than 2 years of experience as a nurse. They served a 12-month tour in Vietnam like all soldiers stationed there and typically worked six 12-hour days per week. Along with their assigned days on duty caring for military personnel, the Army nurses in Vietnam chose to continue to provide medical assistance to the Vietnamese civilians during their off hours. They conducted clinics where basic care could be administered, implemented sick calls at local orphanages, and led classes on child care for the residents of area villages (Norman, 1990).

The nurses stationed in Vietnam treated far more disease-related cases than battlefield injuries, specifically malaria, viral hepatitis, skin diseases, fevers, and diarrheal illnesses. Battlefield injuries were most often the result of assault rifles, rocket-propelled grenades, and booby traps. Multiple wounds tended to be seen when rapid-fire weapons were used. Blasts from mines resulted in severe injuries that were contaminated with debris and shrapnel, setting the stage for horrific infections. However, along with more traumatic injuries, the Vietnam era nurses also were witness to new advances in the treatment of casualties. Rapid evacuation by air, the availability of whole blood, well-established field hospitals, and advanced surgical techniques all combined to generate a mortality rate of 2.6% per thousand patients compared with the 4.5% experienced during World War II.

Vietnam era nurses were renowned for their creativity and ability to improvise equipment in the harshest of conditions: weights were made for traction by wrapping rocks in a Red Cross bag, a drinking straw was made from a piece of plastic gastrointestinal tubing, examination tables were built from discarded scrap lumber, and colostomy bags were formed from plastic dressing wrappers. Such ingenuity allowed the nurses to provide care for thousands of patients under the worst circumstances until the final Army nurse left the Republic of Vietnam in March 1973 (Norman, 1990).

Role Evolution in Modern Nursing

The LPN-to-RN student is one who is already seeking to assume a new role in the healthcare community, and as healthcare reform continues to make sweeping changes in modern medicine and the ways nursing care is delivered, such a student may find that he or she is in a position to not only assume a new role but to tailor that role to his or her own specifications. For example, the American Association of Colleges of Nursing (AACN; 2005) favors requiring nurses who choose to become *advanced practice nurses* such as nurse practitioners, nurse midwives, or certified registered nurse anesthetists to acquire a clinical doctorate, thus allowing them to be referred to as *doctor of nursing practice* (DNP). According to the AACN, such a degree will allow practitioners who have acquired the degree to be on the same professional level as other disciplines, such as audiology, dentistry, medicine, pharmacy, physical therapy, and

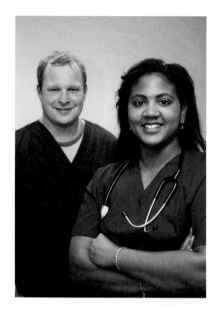

psychology, that have already required a practice doctorate for entry into practice as a health professional. However, the degree is not without controversy; the American Medical Association has expressed great concern regarding the requirement of a clinical doctorate that could potentially allow these advanced practice nurses to uses the title of "doctor" (Miller, 2008).

Although the DNP may open new career avenues for nurses who are interested in a practice-focused doctorate, nurses who obtain such a degree and attempt to teach at the college level may find it difficult to obtain a faculty position and also to acquire a permanent status because the PhD rather than the DNP is considered to be the ultimate degree at such an instructional level (Apold, 2008). Because of such controversy, the usefulness of the DNP to nursing as a profession and to the individual nurse seeking to further his or her career in the 21st century remains to be seen.

The *clinical nurse leader* (CNL) is another nursing role that may play a part in implementing healthcare reform. Initially, in 2003 the AACN proposed the CNL role as a way of responding to the increasing level of care required by the public and the changes in the healthcare environment. The CNL is intended to be capable of leading in all settings of healthcare delivery but is not intended to be an administrative or management position. The CNL is accountable for the healthcare outcomes for a specific set of clients through the use of nursing practice based on clinical research and is capable of functioning both as a provider and manager of care. The CNL may be called on to coordinate, delegate, or supervise care that is provided by the healthcare team (AACN, 2007).

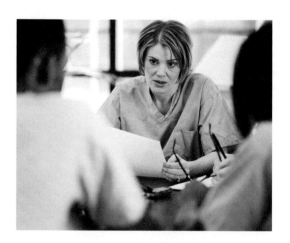

The CNL role requires a thorough understanding of fiscal management, allowing the nurse to effectively manage resources, whether human, environmental, or material. He or she must be able to understand how to manage the budget for a nursing unit as well as how to develop a marketing plan and how to function in an organization (AACN, 2007). Measurement of the performance of the CNL will be determined by the extent to which this nurse can improve both clinical outcomes and cost outcomes for clients.

Summary of Key Points in Chapter

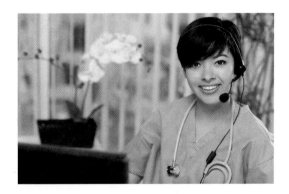

This chapter described the historical development of nursing as a profession. Important concepts and individuals discussed are as follows:

< Edwin Smith Surgical Papyrus
< Provisions of the Mosaic Law and modern nursing
< Contribution of deaconesses and widows to development of modern nursing
< Florence Nightingale
< Dorothea Dix
< Clara Barton
< Sally Louisa Tompkins
< Kate Cumming
< New England Hospital for Women and Children
< Linda Richards
< Mary Eliza Mahoney

In addition, the efforts of nurses during wartime to care for patients were discussed, specifically in relation to World War I, World War II, and the Vietnam War. The evolution of the new roles of DNP and CNL and their relationship to the nursing community were discussed as well.

Conclusion

Like many professions, the history of nursing has been a lengthy one, stretching from Biblical times until the present day (**Figure 1-1**), where it continues to evolve. However, unlike other professions, it has played a part in literally every nation's development because of the universal need for well-being, the desire to be nurtured in a wholesome environment, and the importance of healing of body, mind, and spirit in an environment of safety and security. Nurses will continue to fulfill these needs for humankind worldwide as we move beyond the 21st century.

Communication is a vital part of the healing process that has always characterized nursing. Communication occurs primarily with the patient but also

FIGURE 1-1 Timeline of Significant Events in Nursing History

17th Century

1633: Daughters of Charity of Saint Vincent de Paul founded

↓

1645: North America's first hospital established

↓

18th–19th Century (1830s–1850s)

1836: Nursing Society of Philadelphia founded

↓

1844: Dorothea Dix testified before New Jersey legislature regarding inadequate treatment of the mentally ill; Florence Nightingale traveled to the Institute of Deaconesses at Kaiserworth Germany to be trained as a nurse

↓

1850: School for Nurses opened by Nursing Society of Philadelphia; Florence Nightingale began nurse's training at Institute of St. Vincent de Paul in Alexandria, Egypt

↓

1853: Crimean War broke out; Florence Nightingale visited the Daughters of Charity in Paris for additional training

↓

1854: Florence Nightingale appointed as Superintendent of Crimean War Nursing Staff

↓

(1860s–1870s)

1860: Florence Nightingale published fledgling nursing textbook in the form of *Notes on Nursing: What it is and What it is Not*

↓

1861–1865: American Civil War broke out and American Army Nurses Corp established; Congress authorized women employed as nurses in American Army hospitals for the starting salary of $12/month

↓

1873: Linda Richards graduated from New England Hospital for Women and Children Training School for Nurses and became America's first professional nurse; America's first nursing school based on Nightingale's principles opened at Bellevue Hospital in New York City

↓

1879: Mary Eliza Mahoney graduated from New England Hospital for Women and Children Training School for Nurses and became America's first African-American professional nurse

FIGURE 1-1 **Timeline of Significant Events in Nursing History** *(Continued)*

↓

(1880s–1890s)

1881: Clara Barton became first president of the American Red Cross

↓

1886: First American nursing journal published

↓

1893: Lillian Wald, founder of America's visiting nurses, began teaching home-based nursing classes in New York City; Nightingale Pledge first used by a graduating nursing class at Harper Hospital in Detroit Michigan

↓

1897: American Nurses Association held its first meeting

↓

(1900s–1910s)

1901: New Zealand became first country to regulate nurses nationally

↓

1902: Ellen Dougherty of New Zealand became first registered nurse in the world; Lina Rogers Struthers hired as North America's first school nurse

↓

1908: U.S. Navy Nurse Corp established

↓

1909: University of Minnesota awarded first Bachelors Degree in Nursing

↓

(1920s–1930s)

1923: Yale School of Nursing became first autonomous American school of nursing; Mary Breckinridge founded Frontier Nursing Service

↓

1938: Nurses Memorial in Arlington National Cemetery erected to honor World War I nurses

↓

(1940s and beyond)

1942: U.S. Army nurses imprisoned in the Philippines

↓

1949: U.S. Air Force Nurse Corps established

↓

(Continues)

FIGURE 1-1 **Timeline of Significant Events in Nursing History** *(Continued)*

1956: Columbia University School of Nursing became first American university to grant a Master's Degree in a clinical nursing specialty

↓

1965: First nurse practitioner role established at University of Colorado

↓

1967: Dame Cicely Saunders established first hospice in London

↓

1971: American hospice movement was established

↓

1979: First nursing doctorate established at Case Western Reserve University

Source: AAHN Nursing History Calendar. (2007). Retrieved from American Association for the History of Nursing website: http://www.aahn.org/nursinghistorycalendar.html

---

with family members, the physician, and other caregivers. This process is discussed in the next chapter.

Critical Thinking Questions

1. Review the dietary and hygienic teachings that are specific to the Mosaic Law. Which nursing practices used today can be traced back to these instructions?

2. If the instructions of the Mosaic Law specific to dietary and hygienic practices were implemented today, do you believe the result would be successful? Give the rationale for your answer.

3. Review the characteristics of a nurse under Brahmanism in ancient India. Do you believe the modern-day nurse embodies any of these characteristics? If so, which ones?

4. Do you believe the characteristics that were expected of nurses in the Brahmin-dominated society were realistic? Give the rationale for your answer.

5. Review the set of characteristics that were considered to be necessary for a nurse in India after 1500, as well as the characteristics specified for a nurse during the 17th century. Compare them and discuss how they are similar and how they are different.

6. Compare and contrast the contributions of Dorothea Dix, Clara Barton, Sally Louisa Tompkins, and Kate Cummings to nursing during the American Civil War era.

7. Compare and contrast the contributions of Linda Richards and Mary Eliza Mahoney to the development of modern nursing. Do you believe some of the same obstacles these nursing pioneers faced still exist in nursing today? Be able to support your answer.

8. Compare and contrast the contributions of Helen Fairchild and Vivien Bullwinkel to the development of modern nursing. What coping methods do you believe these heroic nurses used to help them practice nursing under such terrible conditions?

Scenarios

1. Florence Nightingale used the outbreak of the Crimean War as an opportunity to take nursing much further along the route to becoming a respectable profession. What do you believe would be needed today to progress nursing further to becoming a profession that is entered equally by both men and women?

2. Compare and contrast the requirements for a nurse in India after 1500 with those specified by Thomas Fuller, as well as those developed by Dorothea Dix. How did they change over that 300-year period of time, and how did they remain relatively unchanged?

3. Develop a set of qualifications to be a nurse in the 21st century. How do your requirements compare with those for an Indian nurse, those developed by Thomas Fuller, and those specified by Dorothea Dix?

4. Consider the hardships faced by nurses during the various wartime theaters of World War II. Do you believe today's modern nurse would be able to cope as well as these nurses did when faced with similar challenges? Be able to support your answer.

5. What preparation do you believe is needed for the modern nurse to be equipped to deal with a prison-of-war situation such as that faced by the nurses on the island of Corregidor during World War II?

6. How do you believe the role of the nurse changed from World War I to World War II? How do you believe the role of the nurse was affected by changes that occurred in modern medicine during this period of time?

7. Create a table that compares the hardships experienced, role(s) served, and circumstances under which nurses provided care in World War I, World War II, and the Vietnam War.

NCLEX® Questions

Using the information you obtained from studying this chapter, go online to complete the following NCLEX®-format review questions.[1] Visit http://go.jblearning.com/terryLPN using the access code in the front cover of your book. This interactive resource allows you to answer each question and instantly review your results. Practice until you can answer at least 75% successfully and then try to improve your score with each successive attempt.

1. Health-related instructions provided to the Israelites by the priestly tribe of the Levites included (select all that apply):
   a. selection of food that was in accordance with dietary requirements
   b. proper treatment of a woman during pregnancy and childbirth
   c. recognizing communicable disease so that the person could be put to death
   d. specific times for work, rest, and sleep during the course of each day

2. Characteristics required of nurses in India during the period in which Brahmanism was practiced included _____ .
   a. skill in caring for women
   b. skill in caring for children
   c. skill in bathing a patient
   d. skill in assisting with surgery

3. "Able to do everything the best way" is most likely considered a characteristic of a nurse during the time of
   a. Thomas Fuller in the 18th century
   b. Brahminism-era India after 1500 B.C.
   c. Theodor Fliedner in the 19th century
   d. Florence Nightingale in the 19th century

4. "Clever in general" is most likely considered a characteristic of a nurse during the time of
   a. Thomas Fuller in the 18th century
   b. Brahminism-era India after 1500 B.C.
   c. Theodor Fliedner in the 19th century
   d. Florence Nightingale in the 19th century

5. The individual who most effectively revived the Order of the Deaconesses was _____.
   a. Dorothea Dix

---

[1] NCLEX and NCLEX-RN are registered trademarks of the National Council of State Boards of Nursing, Inc.

b. Florence Nightingale

c. Theodor Fliedner

d. Clara Barton

6. Florence Nightingale cared for wounded and dying soldiers during which war or military campaign?

   a. American Civil War

   b. Spanish-American War

   c. World War I

   d. Crimean War

7. The superintendent of female nurses for the Union Army during the Civil War was _____.

   a. Dorothea Dix

   b. Florence Nightingale

   c. Kate Cumming

   d. Clara Barton

8. "Matronly with a serious personality" is a requirement for a female nurse from the set of qualifications developed by _____.

   a. Dorothea Dix

   b. Florence Nightingale

   c. Kate Cumming

   d. Clara Barton

9. The American Red Cross was organized by _____.

   a. Sally Louisa Tompkins

   b. Kate Cumming

   c. Clara Barton

   d. Dorothea Dix

10. The woman who founded a hospital and became appointed as captain of cavalry during the Civil War was

    a. Sally Louisa Tompkins

    b. Kate Cumming

    c. Clara Barton

    d. Dorothea Dix

11. The first trained nurse in America is known to be
    a. Ednah Dow Cheney
    b. Linda Richards
    c. Mary Eliza Mahoney
    d. Helen Fairchild

12. The nurse who became known as the first African-American trained nurse was
    a. Ednah Dow Cheney
    b. Linda Richards
    c. Mary Eliza Mahoney
    d. Helen Fairchild
    e. The nurses who coped with wounded transported on trains known as "moving hospitals" were most likely to have served in which wartime era?
    f. Civil War
    g. World War I
    h. World War II
    i. Vietnam War

13. Helen Fairchild is most closely associated with which era of wartime nursing?
    a. Civil War
    b. World War I
    c. World War II
    d. Vietnam War

14. A nurse who joined the Navy Nurse Corps when it was newly established was most likely to have served during which era of wartime nursing?
    a. Civil War
    b. Vietnam War
    c. World War II
    d. World War I

15. A nurse who was a member of the WAVES was most likely to have served during which era of wartime nursing?
    a. Civil War
    b. Vietnam War
    c. World War II
    d. World War I

16. The World War II era nurse who was the first Army nurse to receive the Purple Heart was
    a. Vivien Bullwinkel
    b. Annie G. Fox
    c. Mildred Clark
    d. Anna May Hays
17. The nurse who became the first nurse in American military history to attain general officer rank was
    a. Vivien Bullwinkel
    b. Annie G. Fox
    c. Mildred Clark
    d. Anna May Hays
18. The doctor of nursing practice degree can most accurately be described as
    a. an administrative or management position requiring knowledge of fiscal management
    b. preparation for the nurse to lead in all settings of healthcare delivery
    c. a clinical doctorate most likely used by an advanced practice nurse
    d. the ultimate degree for a nurse who wishes to provide instruction at the college level
19. The clinical nurse leader role can most accurately be described as
    a. an administrative or management position requiring knowledge of fiscal management
    b. preparation for the nurse to lead in all settings of healthcare delivery
    c. a clinical doctorate most likely used by an advanced practice nurse
    d. the ultimate degree for a nurse who wishes to provide instruction at the college level

For more information on the topics in this chapter and others, please see Appendix on p. 299 for a list of web links to additional resources.

References

American Association of Colleges of Nursing (AACN). (2005). Understanding the doctor of nursing practice (DNP): Evolution, perceived benefits and challenges. Retrieved from http://www.aacn.nche.edu/DNP/dnpfaq.htm

American Association of Colleges of Nursing (AACN). (2007). White paper on the education and role of the clinical nurse leader. Retrieved from http://www.aacn.nche.edu/Publications/WhitePapers/ClinicalNurseLeader.htm

Apold, A. (2008). The doctor of nursing practice: Looking back, moving forward. *Journal for Nurse Practitioners, 4*(2), 101–107.

Barton, C. (1904). *A Story of the Red Cross.* New York, NY: Appleton and Company.

Bellafaire, J. A. (2003). The Army Nurse Corps in World War II. Retrieved from http://www.history.army.mil/books/wwii/72-14/72-14.HTM

Carnegie, M. (1986). *Path We Tread: Blacks in Nursing.* Philadelphia, PA: Lippincott, Wilkins, and Williams.

Doherty, M. (2000). *Letters from Belsen 1945: An Australian Nurse's Experiences with the Survivors of War.* St. Leonards, Australia: NSW College of Nursing.

Donahue, M. P. (1996). *Nursing: The finest art* (2nd ed.). St. Louis, MO: Mosby.

Engle, R., Jr. (1980). Medical center archives. In New York Hospital Training School for Nurses (Cornell University-New York Hospital School of Nursing). Retrieved from http://www.med.cornell.edu/archives/history/timeline.html?name1=Historical+Timeline&type1=2Active

Hagerman, K. (1996). *Dearest of Captains: A Biography of Sally Louisa Tompkins.* Richmond, VA: Bradylane Publishing.

Hilde, L. (2009). Kate Cumming. *Encyclopedia of Alabama.* Retrieved from http://www.encyclopediaofalabama.org/face/ Article.jsp?id=h-1101

Metropolitan State College of Denver. (2004). Women in the military (military life). *The Women Army Corps.* Retrieved from http://www.mscd.edu/history/camphale/wim_001.html

Miller, J. (2008). The doctor of nursing practice: Recognizing a need or graying the line between doctor and nurse? *Medscape Journal of Medicine, 10*(11), 253.

Moses, A. (2011). St. Paula of Rome. *The Self-Ruled Antiochian Orthodox Christian Archdiocese of North America.* Retrieved from http://www.antiochian.org/node/17350

Norman, E. (1990). *Women at War: The Story of Fifty Military Nurses Who Served in Vietnam.* Philadelphia, PA: University of Pennsylvania.

Patrick, B. K. (2011). Army Nurse Helen Fairchild. *Military.com.* Retrieved from http://www.military.com/Content/MoreContent?file=ML_fairchild_bkp

Reiskind, M. (1995). Hospital Founded by Women for Women. *Jamaica Plain Historical Society.* Retrieved from http://www.jphs.org/victorian/hospital-founded-by-women-for-women.html

Schreiber, C. (1999). World War I nurses volunteer for service. *NurseWeek World War I.* Retrieved from http://www.nurseweek.com/features/99-12/ww1.html

Tour Egypt. (2010). The Edwin Smith Surgical Papyrus. Retrieved from http://www.touregypt.net/edwinsmithsurgical.htm

Wentz, A. (1936). *Fliedner the Faithful.* Minneapolis, MN: Board of Publication of the United Lutheran Church in America.

For a full suite of assignments and additional learning activities, use the access code located in the front of your book to visit this exclusive website: http://go.jblearning.com/terryLPN. If you do not have an access code, you can obtain one at the site.

CHAPTER OBJECTIVES

At the end of this chapter, you will be able to:

1. Describe the various elements involved in the process of communication.

2. Diagram a model of the communication process.

3. Discuss the various modes and channels of communication that can be used.

4. Describe various techniques found to be particularly effective and ineffective in communicating verbally with patients.

5. Discuss strategies for communicating effectively with subordinates, physicians, peers, and upper-level management.

KEY TERMS

active listening
channel of communication
communication
decoding
diagonal communication
downward communication
encoding
external climate

grapevine
horizontal communication
incongruent message
I-SBAR-R technique
internal climate
listening
message
mode of communication

nontransactional
    conversation
nonverbal communication
receiver
sender
upward communication
verbal communication

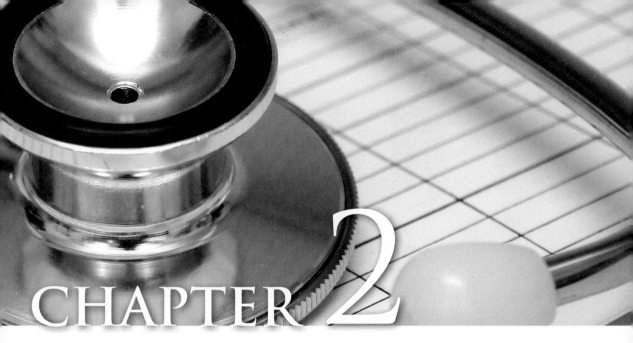

CHAPTER 2

Communication as a Registered Nurse

Introduction to the Communication Process

The process of communication affects every aspect of nursing. Failure to communicate adequately can result in patient injuries, fatalities, and litigation. Marquis and Huston (2012) referred to communication as the most critical leadership skill for the registered nurse (RN) who is moving into the nurse leader or nurse manager role. A RN is required to communicate with a wide variety of individuals daily, including patients, nurse colleagues, superiors such as the nursing supervisor, and subordinates such as nursing assistants. In the 21st century with the advent of e-mail, cellular telephones, and sophisticated computer technology this communication is more complex. A statement that may seem very straightforward when spoken aloud may be completely misconstrued when written as an e-mail. The ability to communicate both clearly and effectively is a prerequisite to the RN moving forward into a leadership role as the next rung on the career ladder (Marquis & Huston, 2012).

Process of Communication

Marquis and Huston (2012) referred to *communication* as an exchange of information that can occur through speech, writing, signals, or behavior. This exchange of information may mean completely different things for the sender of the message and the receiver, and the verbal and nonverbal messages may seem to be completely disconnected.

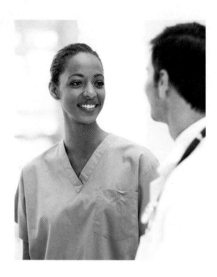

Although communication is a complex, multilayered process, certain elements are necessary in order for it to occur:

< Sender
< Receiver
< Message
< Mode of communicating the message
< Encoding the message
< Decoding the message
< Internal climate of the sender
< External climate of the sender
< Internal climate of the receiver
< External climate of the receiver

For communication to occur there must be at least one *sender*, one *receiver*, and one *message* as well as a *mode* of communicating the message, such as nonverbal, verbal, telephone, or written (**Figure 2-1**). *Encoding* occurs if the sender translates his or her ideas into actual language. *Decoding* occurs as the receiver interprets the message in an attempt to make it meaningful (Finkelman, 2012). The *internal climate* exists for both the sender and the receiver and consists of the person's values, feelings, personality or temperament, and the stress levels under which the message is sent. The *external climate* also exists for both the sender and the receiver and consists of the weather conditions, temperature, timing, and overall organizational climate of the facility in addition to the status of the person involved, his or her level of power, and the degree of authority wielded. Both sender and receiver must be aware of the internal and external climates of the communication process because the

FIGURE 2-1 Model of the Communication Process

SENDER	MESSAGE	RECEIVER
(internal climate/ external climate)	(written, nonverbal, verbal)	(internal climate/ external climate)

Source: Marquis and Huston, 2012.

perception of the message can change drastically if the climate(s) under which the message is sent changes by the time the message is received. Ultimately, for communication to occur effectively, the sender must verify and confirm what the sender saw and heard as his or her version of the received message (Marquis & Huston, 2012).

Modes and Channels of Communication

For a message to be sent a mode of communication must be used (Figure 2-1). As the sender of the message, the RN will need to select the mode based on the circumstances surrounding the message. As the receiver of the message, the RN will interpret the meaning of the message based partially on the mode of communication used. For example, the written mode has the advantage of literally documenting the exact wording of the message. However, it usually requires more time and considerable skill on the part of the nurse. The RN must have polished writing skills to use this mode of communication clearly to avoid being misinterpreted (Marquis & Huston, 2012).

In comparison, the verbal mode of communication can occur more rapidly but does not allow for the documentation that occurs with the written mode. Also, the verbal mode can allow for subtle nuances of speech and voice intonation not possible with other modes. A variation on this mode is telephone communication, but because the receiver cannot observe the sender's facial expression or body language, the message may be more difficult to interpret. This mode of communication is very dependent on environmental conditions and the mechanical structure of the telephone wiring in order for an intact message to be sent (Marquis & Huston, 2012).

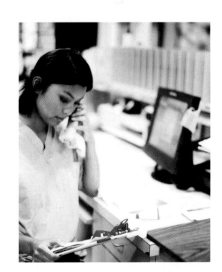

In addition, communication can be nonverbal. This is considered to be the most complex mode in many ways because it includes facial expressions, body movements, and gestures and also communicates the sender's emotional state. As a potential nurse leader, the RN should try to make *nonverbal communication* consistent with *verbal communication*; otherwise, the message can be easily misinterpreted (Marquis & Huston, 2012).

Just as a mode of communication is selected for a message, the RN will choose a *channel of communication* for it as well. See **Table 2-1**. The channel of communication is the direction

TABLE 2-1 **Comparison of Channels of Communication**

Channel	Description	Example
upward	message is sent to a higher level	nurse manager sends message to the nursing supervisor
downward	message is sent to subordinates	nurse manager discusses a situation with staff nurses
horizontal	interaction occurs with others on the same level	nurse manager interacts with other nurse managers in the organization
diagonal	interaction occurs with members of other departments	nurse manager interacts with other department managers in the organization
grapevine	informal, message tends to be distorted, may involve several people simultaneously	hospital's informal information network through which employees may hear erroneous information

in which the message is routed to receivers. For example, when the channel selected is *upward communication*, the RN sends the message to a receiver at a higher level, such as the nursing supervisor. If the channel selected is *downward communication*, the RN sends the message to subordinates, such as when a nurse manager discusses a situation with the staff nurses. The channel of *horizontal communication* is selected when the RN sends a message to others in the organization on the same level as himself or herself. This is used when a nurse manager discusses an issue with other nurse managers from other units in the hospital (Marquis & Huston, 2012).

A variation of this is *diagonal communication*, which occurs when the RN interacts with members of other departments in the facility. This could occur when the Director of Nursing discusses the stocking of a particular medication with the Pharmacy Manager. Although the Pharmacy Manager would not necessarily be at a higher level than the Director of Nursing or have authority over him or her, each recognizes the other as being vital to the functioning of the organization. Finally, the *grapevine* is considered to be the most informal channel of communication. It moves rapidly and may involve several people simultaneously with no discernible systematic route. The message tends to be distorted as it moves throughout the organization's informal network. Because of the tendency for information to be reported erroneously when the grapevine channel is used, the RN who is a nurse leader must continuously stay abreast of the messages that are moving along this bumpy "information highway" and the personnel that contribute to it (Marquis & Huston, 2012).

Verbal Communication in Nursing

Effective communication in nursing, in its verbal form, is especially important because of its influence on the development of an accurate diagnosis of the patient and the selection of appropriate treatment regimen and its significance to patients, as stated on satisfaction surveys. Elliott and Wright (1999) interviewed former patients who had been seriously ill and found that these individuals described that they heard, comprehended, and responded emotionally to verbal communication even when health professionals assumed they could not understand the communication. These patients reported that they found comfort in having caring words addressed to them, particularly when the sender was attempting to communicate with them as one individual to another.

Macdonald (2001) identified several factors that spotlight the importance of communication by nurses, particularly verbal communication:

< Accurate interviewing skills by nurses can produce accurate problem identification.
< Effective communication allows the patient to be cared for as an individual rather than as a collection of symptoms.
< When communication occurs effectively and accurate information is given to patients, research has shown that compliance with drug and treatment regimens tends to increase and patients tend to experience a decrease in stress, pain, and anxiety levels.

The importance of effective interviewing skills on the part of nurses cannot be emphasized enough. When the RN uses a more conversational and exploratory approach to interviewing the patient, the interaction becomes more client-focused and less controlling than the traditional closed-ended, question-and-answer format. An exploratory approach allows the patient the freedom to expand the topics being discussed or even change to a different one entirely. Such interviewing becomes particularly effective when the RN summarizes the patient's verbalized thoughts and feelings periodically, thus demonstrating understanding on the part of the RN, keen interest in the patient's priorities, and a desire to actively discuss these topics with him or her.

Various verbal techniques have been found to be particularly effective when RNs communicate with patients:

- Use open directive questions, such as "How are you coping with the effects of the medication?"
- Use both focusing and clarification simultaneously, such as "You said you have had a great deal of anxiety lately. Please tell me more about the issues with which you are particularly concerned."
- Use empathy and summarizing simultaneously, such as "I sense you are concerned about more issues than only your son's surgery."

Conversely, specific verbal techniques have been found to be especially ineffective in working with patients because they tend to inhibit complete disclosure:

- Use of leading questions, such as "You're feeling better after that pain medication, aren't you?"
- Use of closed-ended questions that only require the patient to answer "yes" or "no," such as "Are you ready to sit up for awhile?"
- Use of advice and reassurance, such as "I'm sure the diagnosis won't be cancer."

Table 2-2 summarizes effective and ineffective communication techniques.

TABLE 2-2 **Effective and Ineffective Verbal Communication Techniques**

Technique	Effective/ Ineffective	Example
Open directive question	effective	"How are you coping with the effects of the medication?"
Simultaneous focusing and clarification	effective	"You said that you have had a great deal of anxiety lately. Are there certain issues that you have been particularly concerns about?"
Simultaneous empathy and summarizing	effective	"I sense that you are concerned about more issues than only your son's surgery."
Leading questions	ineffective	"You're feeling better after that pain medication, aren't you?"
Advice/reassurance	ineffective	"I'm sure that the diagnosis won't be cancer."

Nonverbal Communication in Nursing

Nonverbal communication that occurs between the RN and the patient can be particularly effective and therapeutic. O'Baugh, Wilkes, Sneesby, and George (2009) found that nurses caring for cancer patients who were undergoing chemotherapy treatments frequently used eye contact, therapeutic touching, body movements, and facial expressions while interacting with patients. Smiling was used frequently during the interaction along with humor in an attempt to relax patients during the chemotherapy procedure. The use of therapeutic touch by nurses is particularly significant because it has been shown to decrease stress levels, anxiety, and fatigue in patients undergoing particularly grueling procedures and treatments such as chemotherapy (O'Baugh et al., 2009). In addition, nurses can use observation of nonverbal behavioral cues and facial expressions such as grimacing, clenching and wringing hands, and systematic eye blinking by the patient to know when the individual requires additional pain medication (Shipley, 2010).

A poorly understood aspect of nonverbal communication is *listening*. Consisting of multiple aspects, including empathy, silence, paying attention to the sender's verbal and nonverbal messages, and tolerance and acceptance, it may well be the oldest skills related to caregiving. Empathy involves being aware of and sensitive to the feelings, thoughts, and experiences of another person, in this case the patient. Empathy is needed to help the nurse perceive the patient's experiences (Shipley, 2010).

Silence can be frightening for the task-oriented health professional who wants to take action to solve the patient's problem. However, the importance of silence should not be underestimated because its use gives the patient the time and the permission to communicate as needed without fear of being interrupted with unwanted advice and hollow reassurances. The ability to pay attention to both verbal and nonverbal communication as part of the overall listening experience means the nurse is attentive to both the verbal and nonverbal messages sent by the patient and recognizes when they are incongruent (Shipley, 2010).

Paying attention to tone of voice and body language can increase the nurse's degree of empathy, because both help convey the perception of the patient. All previously discussed aspects of listening include the nurse's ability to be nonjudgmental and accepting. This is necessary for the patient to experience a safe environment in which he or she feels secure enough to communicate thoughts and feelings that have gone unexpressed (Shipley, 2010).

The patient is a multifaceted individual who may have a completely different system of cultural beliefs or a lifestyle that is foreign to the nurse. Listening in a nonjudgmental manner allows the nurse to acknowledge this while simultaneously conveying to the patient that there is no need to fear rejection simply because this difference is present. The nurse must actively choose to lay aside all previously held prejudices and preconceived ideas about the belief system of the patient. Without well-honed listening skills, the nurse cannot use reflection and summarization or provide feedback to the patient to convey the message was communicated and understood (Shipley, 2010).

E-mail

Whereas once written communication in nursing primarily occurred through documentation in a patient's chart, now it can also occur in the form of e-mail. Such a form of communication carries with it its own policies and procedures unique to the healthcare facility as well as various regulations, not the least of which is HIPAA (the Health Insurance Portability and Accountability Act), tied to confidentiality and legal issues. Patient names and other types of identifying information should not be used, and diligence should be maintained in guarding passwords, particularly on the part of licensed individuals such as the RN, who could be subject to discipline by the state board of nursing for violation of patient confidentiality.

E-mail can be used very effectively to document a verbal conversation that was held earlier, to verify points, clarify any inconsistencies, and summarize the primary result of the conversation. As with any form of communication, it is imperative to observe the socially acceptable guidelines for using it, or in this case, the "netiquette" that is appropriate. Such "netiquette" rules are as follows (Finkelman, 2012):

< Indicate if a message is urgent or high priority and also request a return receipt.
< Specify a subject in the subject line; otherwise, the receiver may assume it is irrelevant.
< Ask before attaching sensitive documents such as contracts to an e-mail; the receiver may prefer a hard copy mailed to him or her.
< Do not use abbreviations and symbols in business e-mails because they tend to make such a communication seem less important.
< Begin the e-mail by putting the most important information first; bullets or numbering may be used to highlight highest priority points.

< Be cautious when using color in an e-mail message because some colors may not show up well on a screen.

< When opting to forward a message to another user, include only the most relevant information. Consider if the original sender intended the message to be seen by communicators other than the original receiver.

< When replying to a message, verify that a return communication should be sent only to one recipient rather than as a group reply.

< Verify that messages are received by either requesting a delivery and/or read receipt.

< If an attachment is sent along with a message, verify that the correct attachment is included before sending the message.

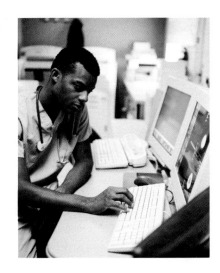

< Do not capitalize every word of a message, because this equates to shouting at the recipient.

< Check spelling and grammar before sending any e-mail communication.

Incongruent Communication

Communications that involve both verbal and nonverbal content and use multiple modes and/or channels during the process of sending the message have the potential to be incongruent. An *incongruent message* is one in which the verbal communication does not seem to match the nonverbal message. What should the RN do when incongruent messages seem to be sent? When the patient clearly is communicating one message verbally and a different message nonverbally, the nurse must be on the alert for signals that the patient is ready to provide additional information to clarify the confusing message. The nurse can then make him- or herself available for the patient to talk more openly. For example, the following conversation between a nurse and a patient contains incongruent communication:

> **RN:** (begins changing bed linen) How are you feeling this morning, Mrs. Smith?
>
> **Patient:** (depressed facial expression) Oh, I think I'm feeling a little better.
>
> **RN:** Did the pain medication help you rest last night?
>
> **Patient:** (turning head to look out of the window of her room) I think so. I woke up early this morning, though. I could hear the change of shift when everyone came in around 6 A.M.
>
> **RN:** I am so sorry you were disturbed! I'll have to caution everyone about being more quiet as they pass by your door early in the morning.

> **Patient:** (looks down at her hands as she winds a paper napkin around her fingers; speaking in a barely audible voice) That's all right. I don't want to be a bother to anyone.
>
> **RN:** (stops changing bed linen and comes to sit down in chair beside patient's bed) Mrs. Smith, I get the feeling that you don't really feel too well today. Can you tell me about your concerns?
>
> **Patient:** (turns to look at RN with a distressed look on her face) I do have some things that are bothering me, but I'm really okay. You go ahead and do what you need to today.
>
> **RN:** (makes eye contact with the patient; takes her hand) Mrs. Smith, you are my priority today. I have plenty of time. You go right ahead and tell me what's bothering you and I'll try my best to help you.

In analyzing the conversation, it becomes clear the patient, although repeatedly reassuring the nurse that she felt better and had no pressing issues, did in fact have some concerns significant enough to disturb her sleep pattern. The nurse avoided giving the patient false reassurance by telling her truthfully that she was a priority and that the nurse would make every effort to help her. Notice the nurse did not give blanket statements that would be interpreted as false reassurances, such as "I'm sure everything will be fine." Such statements are rightfully interpreted by the patient as evidence that the nurse either does not know how to discuss sensitive issues with the patient or does not see such interaction as being a priority.

Barriers to Communication

Several barriers can make the communication process difficult at best and potentially impossible (Finkelman, 2012) (**Table 2-3**):

- *Failing to listen* to the other person involved in the communication can result in negative feelings and responses. This problem can be resolved by practicing ***active listening***, in which the hearer recognizes and acknowledges the person sending the message is conveying an important transmission, whether the receiver agrees with it or not.
- *Practicing selective hearing* occurs when the receiver fails to recognize the needs and problems of the sender. This problem can be resolved by practicing active listening and by making a conscious effort to determine the expectations of the other communicators.
- *Failing to make further inquiries* occurs when the receiver does not request additional information or clarification when the information is vague or confusing. This problem can be resolved by using open-ended questions.

TABLE 2-3 Barriers to Communication

Barrier	Description	Method of Resolution
Failing to listen	Failing to listen to the other person involved in the communication can result in negative feelings and responses being generated.	This problem can be resolved by practicing active listening, in which the hearer recognizes and acknowledges that the person sending the message is conveying an important transmission, whether the receiver agrees with it or not.
Practicing selective hearing	This occurs when the hearer fails to recognize the needs and problems of other individuals communicating.	This problem can be resolved by practicing active listening as well as by making a conscious effort to determine the expectations of the other communicators.
Failing to make further inquiries	This occurs when the person does not request additional information or clarification when the information that he has available is vague or confusing.	This problem can be resolved by using open-ended questions.
Making judgments	This occurs when the receiver decides for himself/herself concerning the overall value of the message.	This problem can be resolved with active listening, making the effort to comprehend other individuals' viewpoints, and pausing before responding.
Expressing opinions while simultaneously practicing intimidation	This effectively prevents any attempt on the part of the other individual communicating from initiating another message.	This problem can be resolved by asking for feedback and consciously being direct rather than aggressive.
Using a defensive approach	Use of a defensive attitude conveys that the communicator does not recognize the value of another point of view.	This problem can be resolved by remaining open to multiple viewpoints that all have value regardless of whether the communicator agrees with them or not.

Barrier	Description	Method of Resolution
Making false inferences	This occurs when the individual communicating decides on a conclusion without having sufficient information to arrive at such a conclusion.	This problem can be resolved by waiting to respond until adequate information has been obtained.
Using personal criticism, profanity, and other types of crude language	This prevents communication by destroying the environment in which the communication is occurring and making the other person communicating uncomfortable.	It can more easily be prevented than resolved through diligent monitoring of one's vocabulary.
Initiating spatial issues	The amount of space between the sender and receiver can create a huge barrier, particularly if one intrudes into the other's personal space and consequently disturbs that person's comfort level.	Such a problem can be prevented more easily than resolved, and this can occur by being mindful of cultural issues related to personal space, space maintained between staff and a particular patient, and the appropriateness of maintaining eye contact.
Maintaining secretiveness	The maintenance of secrecy can be a very destructive practice in terms of communication because of its interference with trust-building and team construction.	This can be resolved through the practice of open communication in which multiple channels of communication are used freely.

< *Making judgments* occurs when the receiver decides for him- or herself about the overall value of the message. This problem can be resolved with active listening, making the effort to comprehend other individuals' viewpoints, and pausing before responding.

< *Expressing opinions while simultaneously practicing intimidation* effectively prevents any attempt on the part of the other individual communicating from initiating another message. This problem can be resolved by asking for feedback and consciously being direct rather than aggressive.

< *Overusing reassurance and/or rejection* effectively stops communication. This problem can be resolved by maintaining open communication

in conjunction with an attitude of respect for the other individual communicating.

< *Using a defensive approach* conveys that the communicator does not recognize the value of another point of view. This problem can be resolved by remaining open to multiple viewpoints that all have value regardless of whether the communicator agrees with them or not.

< *Making false inferences* occurs when the individual communicating decides on a conclusion without having sufficient information to arrive at such a conclusion. This problem can be resolved by waiting to respond until adequate information has been obtained.

< *Using personal criticism, profanity, and other types of crude language* prevents communication by creating an unsafe and uncomfortable environment in which to communicate. It can more easily be prevented than resolved through diligent monitoring of one's vocabulary.

< *Initiating spatial issues* creates an adequate amount of space between the sender and receiver and avoids intrusion into the other's personal space, potentially disturbing that person's comfort level. Such a problem can be prevented more easily than resolved by being mindful of cultural issues related to personal space, the space that is maintained between staff and a particular patient, and both the ability and the appropriateness of maintaining eye contact.

< *Maintaining secretiveness* can be a very destructive practice in terms of communication because of its interference with trust-building and team construction. This can be resolved through the practice of open communication in which multiple channels of communication are used freely.

Active listening consists of being completely focused on the person who is communicating a message. It includes listening without judgment while absorbing the conversation to such an extent that the listener can repeat to the speaker most of what was intended as the meaning. Yoder-Wise (2011) noted some guidelines that can be used to further the process of active listening:

< Do not allow yourself to interrupt the speaker.
< Gain as much information as possible through listening to prevent misinterpreting the speaker's meaning.
< The speaker's first words may not necessarily represent his or her genuine thoughts and feelings, so you'll need to listen closely to determine the true meaning of the communication.
< As you listen, detach yourself from your own beliefs and views and judgments to understand the perspective of the speaker.

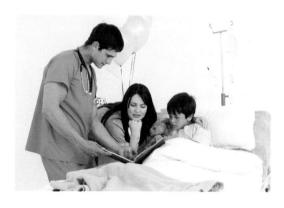

< Recognize that any prejudices you hold will influence you as you listen to the other person.

< Realize that you must first listen to the speaker and understand his or her perspective before determining if you agree with that perspective. Effective listening cannot occur without having a genuine desire to grasp the speaker's perspective.

Once we understand what active listening is, we must then determine how it can be used. Active listening should be used as follows (Yoder-Wise, 2011):

< To convey interest in what the speaker is saying

< To encourage the speaker to expand further on his or her verbalized thoughts

< To help the speaker clarify the problem in his or her own thinking

< To help the speaker hear what he or she has said in the manner in which it sounded to the listener

< To extract key ideas from a long statement or an extended discussion

< To respond to a speaker's feelings more than to his or her verbalization

< To summarize the speaker's points of agreement and disagreement to form a basis for more discussion

< To express a consensus of how a group feels after hearing the speaker

Communication with Peers

Once there is an understanding of the process of communication as well as the various aspects of verbal and nonverbal communication, the RN can begin to examine how he or she communicates with peers, subordinates, physicians, and upper-level management. Communication with peers typically occurs using a horizontal flow of information. This directional flow is due to the equality that is present in the interaction, because no particular person has greater power during the communication. Ideally, there is a sense of trust and respect present and cohesiveness that evolves as nurses work together (Zerwekh & Garneau, 2012).

It is critical that peer communication is accurate when the care of the patient is being transferred to another nurse, such as at the end of a shift, when the patient is having a procedure done, or when the patient is being transferred to another unit of the hospital for care. In these cases it is essential that all aspects of the patient's care be accurately communicated to the nurse accepting care of the patient. The Joint Commission's National Patient Safety Goals now emphasize that a standardized procedure should be used when communicating such vital information to a colleague in such a situation. Referred to as the *I-SBAR-R technique*, the procedure is as follows (Zerwekh & Garneau, 2012):

- I = **Identification:** Identify yourself as the nurse and identify the patient using two methods of identification
- S = **Situation:** Describe what is going on
- B = **Background:** Describe what led to the current situation and the patient's status before this
- A = **Assessment:** Describe what you believe to be happening
- R = **Response/Request:** Describe what you believe should happen
- R = **Readback/Response:** The receiver acknowledges the information that was given and gives a response

The I-SBAR-R technique's importance cannot be overemphasized because it promotes critical-thinking skills by requiring the sender of the communication to assess the patient and design a recommendation before the communication is actually delivered (Zerwekh & Garneau, 2012). It can contribute significantly to a very effective horizontal flow of information during a communication.

Communication with Subordinates

For many RNs who are promoted into a nurse leader role such as the nurse manager, a challenging part of that role can be learning how to communicate effectively with subordinate employees. For effective communication to occur with employees, nurse leaders must be honest with them about whatever situation is the focus at the moment, create an environment of mutual respect, and work toward a gradual development of a strong bond of trust. An easy and often effective way to develop such respect and trust with employees is to informally communicate for a few minutes each day with each person. It may be no more than a brief inquiry regarding the person's elderly parents and their health issues, for example, but such a query will be meaningful to the employee because it signals personalized interest on the part of the nurse leader. This is frequently referred to as *nontransactional conversation*, meaning it is not necessarily intended to have a specific purpose. In addition, if the pace of the nursing unit allows it, the nurse leader may find it particularly effective to meet

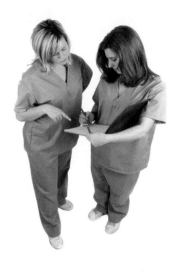

with the administrative staff one layer down, such as the assistant nurse manager, for example, at least weekly to make certain he or she is kept up-to-the-minute with developing issues (Belzer-Riley, 2007).

It is also important to recognize the good work of employees, to counter any criticism that must be leveled with positive comments, and to thank employees for their contribution to a project, if possible, publicly. It is particularly important to recognize the significance that unspoken signals can have for subordinate employees. For example, calling an employee into your office to discuss a problem with him or her emphasizes the difference in the power distribution in the relationship and may affect the dynamics of the interaction that ensues. In comparison, going to an employee's office emphasizes the collegiality that is present in the relationship and may lead to a more open and positive exchange of information even if the communication primarily centers around a problem that has developed (Belzer-Riley, 2007).

One of the most important aspects of communicating with subordinate employees is making the commitment to active listening. This can be implemented with employees through use of several strategies:

< Develop a mechanism for formal feedback: This can be something as simple as a suggestion box. If possible, ensure anonymity so employees will be more open and honest and can approach you with situations that might not be brought to your attention otherwise.
< Give serious attention to the information provided by employees: Employees recognize if you use their suggestions and information. If suggestions from employees are never used, at some point they will stop and the nurse leader will find that a previously busy information superhighway has become a one-way street.
< Reward suggestions that are used or feedback that is particularly useful: Design some type of reward for employees who take the initiative to make suggestions that help the overall functioning of the nursing unit or that allow the provision of more effective, higher quality patient care.

Just as active listening has been shown to be an invaluable tool in communicating with patients, it is equally effective to the nurse leader who is communicating with subordinate employees (Belzer-Riley, 2007).

Communication with Physicians

For many nurses communicating with physicians can be the most difficult part of their daily patient care routine. Nadzam (2009) attributed this difficulty to different communication styles, as nurses are trained to communicate in a manner that is both narrative and descriptive, whereas physicians are trained to communicate in an action-oriented manner that requires immediate attention. The following communication barriers between physicians and nurses have been identified (Nadzam, 2009):

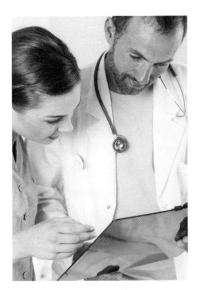

- A lack of structure, policies, and procedures related to verbal reports in terms of content, timing, or purpose of the reports
- A lack of a shared mental model for verbal healthcare communication
- A lack of rules for verbal transmission of information, whether by face-to-face or by telephone
- Difference of opinion among healthcare professionals regarding what type of information should be communicated during a verbal report
- Frequent interruptions and disruptions
- Frequency with which communication occurs

Merely recognizing that such barriers exist is not a solution to ensuring satisfactory communication between physicians and nurses. The Joint Commission now requires all healthcare organizations to take steps to improve the effectiveness of communication that occurs between all caregivers, including physicians and nurses, as part of its National Patient Safety Goals (The Joint Commission, 2011). These measures include developing a list of unacceptable abbreviations and reporting critical test results within a specified timeframe.

Furthermore, healthcare organizations are responsible for ensuring that important information regarding a patient's condition is consistently transferred from one caregiver to the next oncoming caregiver. In addition, specific strategies have been noted to help improve the communication that occurs between nurses and physicians (Nadzam, 2009):

- The nurse should address the physician by name.
- The nurse should have patient information and the chart readily available before attempting to contact the physician.
- The nurse should clearly verbalize any concern regarding the patient as well as the reasons leading to such concern; the physician should recognize such verbalized concern as being valid and worthy of consideration.
- The nurse should develop a potential appropriate follow-up plan; the physician should be prepared to consider such a plan.

< The nurse should focus on the patient's problem when communicating with the physician rather than any extenuating circumstances that may exist; the physician should ensure that sufficient orders are given to deal with the problem at hand.

< Both nurses and physicians should be professional in their demeanor without showing evidence of aggression.

< Both nurses and physicians should monitor the problems of the patient until all such problems either have been resolved in a satisfactory manner or the major exacerbation of chronic disease processes has been eliminated.

Consistent implementation of such strategies may lead to an improvement in the communication that occurs between physicians and nurses.

Communicating with Upper-Level Management

Communication with personnel that serve in a supervisory capacity customarily takes on a formal tone. The message you communicate to your supervisor may well be moved upward along the chain of command to a director of nursing or assistant vice president for nursing, then to a vice president for nursing, and ultimately to the chief executive officer. Therefore, to ensure accurate communication, make your message straightforward without being blunt and courteous without seeming to hedge on making a request (Marquis & Huston, 2012).

When communicating with upper-level management, it is extremely important to be assertive without becoming aggressive by expressing your concerns directly and honestly without interfering with the rights of another individual. The assertive individual is capable of stating his or her views using "I" statements while consciously making verbal and nonverbal communication congruent.

Assertive communication does not include rude or insensitive behavior but does include speaking as an informed member of a profession. What should the assertive RN do when forced to communicate with an aggressive person (Marquis and Huston, 2012)?

< Use reflection: Reflect the speaker's message back to him or her, focusing on affective aspects of the message. This allows the aggressive speaker to

determine if the situation warrants his or her use of such highly charged speech patterns and/or anger. Let the speaker know that you are hearing the message that he or she is sending and are paying attention. For example, when communicating with a patient's irate family member, the RN could state, "I hear you saying that you are more upset about this than you have ever been before."

< Repeat an assertive message: This can be very effective when the aggressor persists in a consistent line of thinking or begins to dramatize the situation. For example, the nurse manager who is interacting with an aggressive vice president for nursing can remark, "I can see that you're very upset about this, and I'd like to discuss this with you, but not here at the nurse's station. Would you prefer to talk in your office or mine?"

< Restate the message assertively: Rephrase the aggressive communicator's message so it is delivered in an assertive manner while eliminating the extreme emotions that were previously included. For example, the nurse manager could say to a physician who becomes aggressive, "I hear you saying that you consider Mr. Doe's care to be your highest priority and we certainly want him to have a positive outcome from his hospitalization as well."

< Pose a question: If the nurse manager is communicating with the vice president for nursing, for example, who is implying that a specific employee may warrant being fired, the nurse manager can assertively ask the vice president if complaints have been received regarding the employee's work performance.

Zerwekh and Garneau (2012) noted guidelines to be used by the RN communicating with a supervisor:

< Keep the supervisor informed of pertinent information on a regular basis. Show a sense of responsibility by gathering important information to share with the supervisor.

< If you detect a problem developing, have specific information ready to give the supervisor with as much documentation gathered as possible; have several possible solutions to the problem already developed and ready for implementation.

< Avoid assigning blame, exaggerating, or using an excessive amount of drama in word choices.

< Do not initiate a conversation when angry, and do not respond to one with anger. Explain your thoughts and feelings on a subject assertively but calmly, using "I" statements.

< Present an idea for a new project to the supervisor in the form of a written proposal that has all necessary information gathered, and then arrange to meet after giving adequate time for the proposal to be read.

< Accept feedback whether positive or negative, and learn from it even if you don't agree with it.

< Follow the chain of command by taking a problem to the supervisor first before going on to the next link in the chain of command. If you try to bypass this step, most likely the person that you approach will ask if you have spoken to your supervisor about the matter and will send you back to speak to the supervisor before you are allowed to move further.

Summary of Key Points in Chapter

The chapter discussed the use of communication by RNs. The various elements involved in the process of communication were described and their position in a model of the communication process were specified, including sender, receiver, ending, and decoding. The various modes and channels of communication were discussed, including verbal and nonverbal communication and upward, downward, diagonal, and horizontal communication. Techniques found to be particularly effective in communicating verbally with patients were described, as well as techniques that have been found to be particularly ineffective in such situations. Finally, strategies were offered to stimulate effective communication with

< Subordinates
< Physicians
< Nursing peers
< Upper-level management

Conclusion

Here we discussed the various types of communication the RN may be called upon to use at various points in his or her career path. Without adequate command of communication skills, sufficient understanding of the process by which communication takes place, and the appropriate type of communication to use in various contexts, the RN runs the risk of not only failing to progress in his or her career but also sabotaging the current rung he or she holds on the career ladder.

Another method by which communication occurs that is specific to nursing is the nursing process. The intricacies of this process are discussed in the next chapter.

Critical Thinking Questions

1. Write down a conversation you recently had with another person and identify how the communication process occurred during the conversation. Identify the sender, the receiver, the internal and external climates of both the sender and receiver (to the extent that you know such information), the message that was sent, and both the mode and channel of communication. Were you able to determine if the message you sent was the same one received? Why or why not?

2. Create a verbal communication between an RN and a patient that uses at least three effective verbal communication techniques.

3. Create a verbal communication between an RN and a patient that requires the nurse to use aspects of listening: empathy, silence, and tolerance and acceptance. How can you as the nurse determine if your listening skills are sufficiently developed as you care for patients?

4. Create a communication between yourself as an RN and another RN in which you use the I-SBAR-R technique. Describe in detail what is communicated as the technique is used, including the response from the other nurse.

5. A newly promoted nurse manager is having difficulty working with an assistant vice president for nursing who tends to communicate in an aggressive manner. Develop at least three communication strategies that could be used effectively in this situation and give examples of verbal communication that would use each of the strategies.

Scenarios

1. You are the unit manager of a 25-bed medical-surgical floor. It has been brought to your attention that the staff members are very anxious because a rumor has been circulating through the "grapevine" that the hospital is to be sold. This is not correct; in fact, the hospital will be expanded, not sold, and an additional 25 nurses will be hired.

   Analyze this situation. How do you believe this channel of communication came to be used for this particular message? Whom do you believe has been contributing to use of this channel? What do you believe would have been a more appropriate channel of communication for the accurate version of this message? Be prepared to give your rationale for your answer.

2. You are the unit manager of a six-bed pediatric intensive care unit. One of your patients is a 12-year-old girl who received second-degree burns throughout most of her body when the family home burned to the ground during the night. During the fire the girl's mother was severely burned and her father was killed. The mother has been transferred to another hospital for specialized treatment for her injuries. The girl seems to be severely depressed and does not interact in any way with staff as they care for her. She has not spoken since her admission to the unit. You arrange a meeting with your staff nurses to discuss techniques to use in communicating with this patient to increase her interaction, both verbal and nonverbal, with the staff. What suggestions do you believe the nurses would have for this patient?

3. You were promoted to the position of nurse manager of a 10-bed cardiac intensive care unit 2 weeks ago. One of the staff nurses comes to see you approximately three times a week with suggestions for ways to improve the functioning of the unit. Another staff nurse tells you that the previous nurse manager never interacted with the subordinate personnel and disliked suggestions. Describe at least three strategies for communicating with each of these nurses.

4. You are a unit manager on the oncology floor. One of your nurses comes to you in tears because she says she cannot work with Dr. Lange, the primary physician for that particular floor. You talk with the rest of the staff and find out that all of them have difficulty at times communicating with the physicians who work with these patients. What do you believe will be the most effective strategies to use in communicating with Dr. Lange and the other physicians?

5. As the unit manager of a 30-bed medical-surgical floor, you have recently hired several new staff members. One of them is Carrie, a 30-year-old RN with 7 years of experience. Her patient skills are excellent, and she has better IV insertion technique than any other nurse on the floor. However, after Carrie has been on staff for 6 weeks, you get complaints from the other nurses as well as the physicians regarding her ability to communicate. Carrie becomes very defensive when a question is asked about her patient care. She normally peppers her speech patterns with profanity and various types of crude remarks. The physicians complain that Carrie does not seem to be listening to them as they give her verbal orders while making rounds. Document a conversation that occurs between you and Carrie in which you have to discuss these problems with her as she ends her probationary period.

NCLEX® Questions

Using the information you obtained from studying this chapter, go online to complete the following NCLEX®-format review questions. Visit http://go.jblearning.com/terryLPN using the access code in the front cover of your book. This interactive resource allows you to answer each question and instantly review your results. Practice until you can answer at least 75% successfully, and then try to improve your score with each successive attempt.

1. The RN analyzes a message's sender to determine the person's values, feelings, personality, and stress level. The nurse is most likely to classify this as the sender's
   a. internal climate
   b. decoding
   c. external climate
   d. encoding

2. The RN analyzes the way in which the sender of a message translates his or her ideas into actual language. The nurse is most likely to classify this as the sender's
   a. internal climate
   b. decoding
   c. external climate
   d. encoding

3. The staff RN who sends a message to the nursing supervisor is most likely using which channel of communication?
   a. upward
   b. downward
   c. horizontal
   d. diagonal

4. The nurse manager who discusses a problem on the nursing unit with the staff RNs is most likely using which channel of communication?
   a. upward
   b. downward
   c. horizontal
   d. diagonal

5. The nurse manager who discusses a problem with the director of pharmacy is most likely using which channel of communication?
   a. upward
   b. downward

    c. horizontal

    d. diagonal

6. When one staff RN discusses a problem with another staff RN on the same unit, the sender of the message is most likely using which channel of communication?

    a. upward

    b. downward

    c. horizontal

    d. diagonal

7. An example of an open direct question an RN could ask a patient is

    a. "How do you feel about your diagnosis?"

    b. "Are you in pain today?"

    c. "Will you need something to help you sleep?"

    d. "Can you rate your discomfort on a 1–10 scale?"

8. An example of a leading question a nurse might ask a patient is

    a. "Do you have anyone at home to help you after surgery?"

    b. "Are you ready to sit up for awhile now?"

    c. "You don't want any more of that juice, do you?"

    d. "How would you describe your childhood?"

9. An example of an RN giving false reassurance to a patient is

    a. "You seem to have a great deal of anxiety related to your surgery."

    b. "How are you coping with the side effects of the chemotherapy?"

    c. "I'm sure that everything will be fine after your surgery."

    d. "Can you show me where you're having discomfort?"

10. Recognizing and acknowledging the sender of a message is conveying an important transmission even if the receiver doesn't agree with it is known as _____.

    a. making judgments

    b. practicing selective hearing

    c. initiating spatial issues

    d. active listening

11. When the receiver of a message decides for himself about the overall value of a message, he is _____.

    a. making judgments

    b. practicing selective hearing

    c. initiating spatial issues

    d. active listening

12. Failing to recognize the needs and problems of other people communicating is known as _____.
    a. making judgments
    b. practicing selective hearing
    c. initiating spatial issues
    d. active listening

13. The elements of the I-SBAR-R technique include
    a. identification, situation, background, assessment, response/request, and readback/response
    b. intervention, situation, background, assessment, response/request, and readback/response
    c. identification, situation, background, assessment, response/request, and repeat/response
    d. implementation, scenario, background, assessment, response/request, and readback/response

14. To improve the communication between nurses and physicians (select all that apply),
    a. the nurse should avoid addressing the physician by name to show respect for him or her
    b. the nurse should have the chart available before the physician is contacted
    c. the nurse should be professional in his or her demeanor without being aggressive
    d. the nurse should develop a follow-up plan that could be suggested if necessary

15. When communicating with an aggressive person, the most appropriate communication technique the RN should use is
    a. leading
    b. clarification
    c. focusing
    d. reflection

16. Communication barriers that may exist between physicians and nurses include (select all that apply)
    a. lack of rules for face-to-face or telephone transmission of information
    b. difference of opinion regarding what information should be included in report
    c. frequent interruption and disruptions occurring during communication

      d. congruence regarding how often communication should occur

17. What should the assertive RN do when communicating with an aggressive person who begins to over-dramatize the situation?
    a. use reflection when speaking
    b. repeat an assertive message
    c. restate message assertively
    d. pose a question

18. What should the assertive RN do to help an aggressive speaker determine if the situation warrants the use of anger?
    a. use reflection when speaking
    b. repeat an assertive message
    c. restate message assertively
    d. pose a question

19. What should the assertive RN do to eliminate the extreme emotions included in an aggressive communicator's message?
    a. use reflection when speaking
    b. repeat an assertive message
    c. restate message assertively
    d. pose a question

20. The RN has a problem that she believes should be addressed by hospital administration. With whom should the RN speak initially to move up the chain of command?
    a. vice president for nursing
    b. chief nursing officer
    c. medical director
    d. nursing supervisor

For more information on the topics in this chapter and others, please see Appendix on p. 299 for a list of web links to additional resources.

References

Belzer-Riley, J. (2007). *Communication in Nursing*. Philadelphia, PA: Mosby.

Elliott, R., & Wright, L. (1999). Verbal communication: What do critical care nurses say to their unconscious or sedated patients? *Journal of Advanced Nursing, 29,* 1412–1420.

Finkelman, A. (2012). *Leadership and management for nurses* (2nd ed.). Boston, MA: Pearson.

Macdonald, L. M. (2001). *Nurse talk: Features of effective verbal communication used by expert district nurses.* Master's thesis, Victoria University, Wellington, New Zealand.

Marquis, B. L., & Huston, C. J. (2012). *Leadership roles and management functions in nursing* (7th ed.). Philadelphia, PA: Lippincott Williams & Wilkins.

Nadzam, D. (2009). Nurses' role in communication and patient safety. *Journal of Nursing Care Quality, 24*(3), 184–187.

O'Baugh, J., Wilkes, L. M., Sneesby, K., & George, A. (2009). Investigation into the communication that takes place between nurses and patients during chemotherapy. *Journal of Psychosocial Oncology, 27,* 396–414.

Shipley, S. D. (2010). Listening: A concept analysis. *Nursing Forum, 45*(2), 125–134.

The Joint Commission. (2011). National Patient Safety Goals. Retrieved from http://www.jointcommission.org/standards_information/npsgs.aspx

Yoder-Wise, P. (2011). *Leading and managing in nursing* (5th ed.). St. Louis, MO: Elsevier.

Zerwekh, J., & Garneau, A. Z. (2012). *Nursing today: Transition and trends* (7th ed.). St. Louis, MO: Elsevier.

For a full suite of assignments and additional learning activities, use the access code located in the front of your book to visit this exclusive website: http://go.jblearning.com/terryLPN. If you do not have an access code, you can obtain one at the site.

CHAPTER OBJECTIVES

At the end of this chapter, you will be able to:

1. Define the nursing process as it is used by the registered nurse.

2. Describe the various steps of the nursing process.

3. Provide examples of the use of the steps of the nursing process in patient care.

4. Describe the various domains of learning as used in Bloom's taxonomy.

5. Document examples of the various types of nursing interventions.

KEY TERMS

affective domain
assessment
Bloom's taxonomy
cognitive domain
dependent nursing
    intervention
domain
emergency assessment
evaluation

focused assessment
independent nursing
    intervention
initial assessment
interdependent nursing
    intervention
nursing goal
nursing diagnosis
nursing process

objective data
ongoing assessment
outcome criteria
planning
psychomotor domain
subjective data
taxonomy

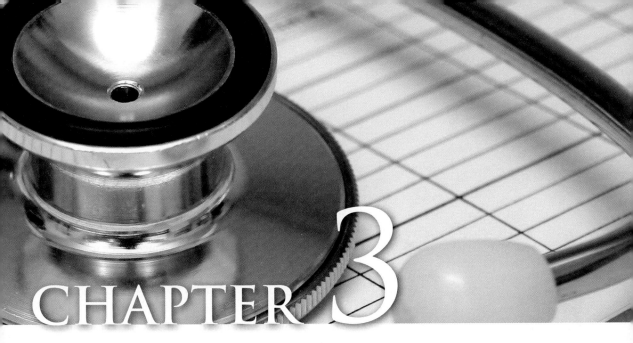

CHAPTER 3

The Nursing Process

Introduction to the Nursing Process

As the registered nurse (RN) functions daily as a nurse leader, he or she will be called on to exercise critical thinking and nursing judgment. The nurse will be required to demonstrate that he or she can effectively collect the various pieces of information about a patient's presenting symptoms, existing disease processes, support system, medication regimen, and psychological state to formulate a plan of nursing care for the patient. The process by which those pieces are collected, scrutinized as to their value, and analyzed regarding their applicability to the patient is known as the *nursing process*. Implementation of the nursing process and its subsequent documentation result in the development of a plan for the nursing care of the patient (Gardner, 2002).

Why is the nursing process important? Above all, it is centered around the patient or client. It requires the nurse to individualize the plan being developed, because a generic plan may well serve as an effective framework for a patient but requires specific changes to be made based on the needs of each patient. The nursing process helps the RN (Gardner, 2002)

< Stay organized during collection of data regarding the patient
< Develop a nursing diagnosis to describe the patient's current situation
< Plan a regimen of nursing care to assist in resolving the patient's problem to the greatest extent possible

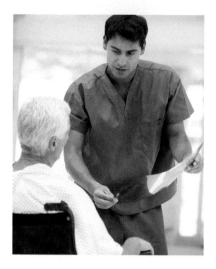

‹ Implement the steps involved in the regimen of nursing care
‹ Evaluate the effectiveness of the care that was carried out

In addition, the nursing process assists the RN in effective use of time management as well as conservation of resources. Those resources may be financial, personnel, or energy. Therefore, the nursing process can lead to effective assessment, so that fewer supplies are charged to the patient; effective planning, so that fewer personnel are required to be assigned to the patient's care; and effective implementation, so that fewer nurses experience physical or emotional exhaustion in caring for a chronically ill patient.

The advantages of the nursing process when used effectively are as follows: (Alfaro-Lefevre, 2009)

‹ To ensure the patient's health concerns and his or her response to them are the focus of the nursing care plan
‹ To ensure care that is planned and implemented is individualized for the patient
‹ To promote the patient's participation in his or her care by encouraging autonomy as the plan is implemented, and to provide the patient with a sense of control rather than the helplessness that can come with long-term assumption of the patient role
‹ To improve communication by providing nurses with a summary of the patient's identified health issues and all current data known about the issues
‹ To require accountability for nursing actions that are implemented; such accountability then promotes delivery of the highest quality health care
‹ To require the use of critical thinking, problem solving, and use of nursing judgment
‹ To focus on the achievement of patient outcomes
‹ To minimize errors that can occur during the delivery of patient care

Assessment

Assessment is arguably the most important step in the nursing process because it involves data collection on the various health issues being experienced by the patient.

Both licensed practical nurses and RNs can contribute to data collection, but only the RN analyzes the data and uses them to formulate a comprehensive assessment of the patient that will ultimately be used in the development of a plan of nursing care (Quan, 2007).

For an assessment to be comprehensive it must be holistic, and this can only occur if the data gathered includes a physical examination and an exhaustive health history. The data gathered through the health history should include subjective data, which is information retrieved from the patient's verbalization, and objective data, which is information retrieved from observation of the patient, including reviewing the results of diagnostic testing. The data gathered through assessment can occur through four variations of this process (**Table 3-1**):

TABLE 3-1 Types of Assessment

Type of Nursing Assessment	Characteristics
initial	This occurs upon initial contact with the patient and is usually as comprehensive as possible. It begins with the symptoms that caused the patient to seek assistance from the healthcare community and should culminate in a head-to-toe view of the patient's level of functioning.
focused	The focused assessment is performed on each problem once they have been identified. This type of assessment is important because it allows symptoms to be examined in greater detail, promotes the weighing of various etiologies to explain those symptoms, searches for contributing factors, and examines patient characteristics that would also help solve the presenting problem or at least clarify the issue. Focused assessment will be initiated again if a new symptom or problem suddenly emerges.
emergency	This is utilized when time is of the essence due to the life-threatening nature of the patient's problem. It will include only essential data that is relevant to the patient's immediate issue. Once the patient's situation is stable and is no longer considered life-threatening, additional data can be gathered.
ongoing	This is considered to be occurring continuously throughout a patient's healthcare experience. Data may be gathered with the assistance of electronic equipment such as may be seen in a critical care unit, and the ongoing assessment usually will include periodic episodes of data-gathering that occur routinely, such as every four hours for vital signs, for example. The interval for such ongoing assessment may be able to be changed at the discretion of the RN, in some cases.

< *Initial assessment*: This occurs on initial contact with the patient and is usually as comprehensive as possible. It begins with the symptoms that caused the patient to seek assistance from the healthcare community and should culminate in a head-to-toe view of the patient's level of functioning (Harkreader, Hogan, & Thobaben, 2007).

< *Focused assessment*: This is performed on each problem once identified. This type of assessment is important because it allows symptoms to be examined in greater detail, promotes the weighing of various etiologies to explain those symptoms, searches for contributing factors, and examines patient characteristics that would also help solve the presenting problem or at least clarify the issue. Focused assessment will be initiated again if a new symptom or problem suddenly emerges.

< *Emergency assessment*: This is used when time is of the essence due to the life-threatening nature of the patient's problem. It includes only essential data relevant to the patient's immediate issue. Once the patient's situation is stable and is no longer considered life-threatening, additional data can be gathered (Harkreader et al., 2007).

< *Ongoing assessment*: This occurs continuously throughout a patient's healthcare experience. Data may be gathered with the assistance of electronic equipment, and the ongoing assessment usually includes periodic episodes of routine data gathering, such as every 4 hours for vital signs. The interval for such ongoing assessment may change at the discretion of the RN, in some cases (Harkreader et al., 2007).

As the RN begins the process of analyzing the data, he or she will find that it can be classified as either subjective or objective. *Subjective data* are information received from the patient because it cannot be observed directly by the nurse. Examples of subjective data include pain, nausea, and dizziness. In comparison, *objective data* are considered to be information about the client obtained through direct observation. This type of data yields information that is measurable. Examples of objective data are blood pressure, pulse, respiration, and temperature readings (Harkreader et al., 2007).

The data comprising the assessment phase of the nursing process can be gathered through physical examination of the patient, observation of the characteristics of the patient's symptoms, review of the results of laboratory and diagnostic tests, discussion with other health professionals, and, most importantly, through interviewing the patient. Such an interview should focus on the patient's chief complaint that led him or her to seek medical assistance and should include a discussion of the patient's past medical history; family medical history' and pertinent religious, cultural, and psychosocial concerns. The interview should include a summary of the important information gleaned from the discussion with the patient (Harkreader et al., 2007).

Diagnosis

Once assessment information has been gathered and analyzed and the RN has begun making decisions about patient care, a nursing diagnosis can be selected. The *nursing diagnosis* is both measurable and realistic and is used to direct the nursing process as it is individualized for the patient. A list of accepted nursing diagnoses was developed by the North American Nursing Diagnosis Association (NANDA, 2011). These diagnoses are classified using a system known as *taxonomy*. The classification system yields 13 domains that are then subdivided into classes and, ultimately, into diagnoses (NANDA, 2011). The domains are as follows:

< Activity/rest
< Circulation
< Ego integrity
< Elimination
< Food/fluid
< Hygiene
< Neurosensory
< Pain/discomfort
< Respiration
< Safety
< Sexuality
< Social interaction
< Teaching/learning

Table 3-2 shows the nursing diagnoses developed by NANDA according to the respective domain.

How is a nursing diagnosis formulated? The diagnosis consists of a problem combined with a primary cause, also referred to as the etiology, if such information is known. Five types of problems may be experienced by the patient (Gardner, 2002) (**Table 3-3**):

1. Actual: This problem
< Is currently experienced by the patient
  < Can be validated by specific symptoms the patient notices along with specific signs observed by the nurse.

TABLE 3-2 **2009–2011 Nursing Diagnoses**
(organized according to nursing focus by Doenges/Moorhouse diagnostic divisions)

ACTIVITY/REST—Ability to engage in necessary/desired activities of life (work and leisure) and to obtain adequate sleep/rest

Activity intolerance, risk for

Activity planning, ineffective disuse syndrome, risk for diversional activity, deficient fatigue

Insomnia, lifestyle, sedentary

Mobility, impaired bed mobility, impaired wheelchair sleep, readiness for enhanced sleep deprivation

Sleep pattern, disturbed transfer ability, impaired walking, impaired

CIRCULATION—Ability to transport oxygen and nutrients necessary to meet cellular needs

Autonomic dysreflexia, risk for

Bleeding, risk for cardiac output, decreased

Intracranial adaptive capacity, decreased

Perfusion, ineffective peripheral tissue

Perfusion, risk for decreased cardiac tissue

Perfusion, risk for ineffective cerebral tissue

Perfusion, risk for ineffective gastrointestinal

Perfusion, risk for ineffective renal

Shock, risk for

EGO INTEGRITY—Ability to develop and use skills and behaviors to integrate and manage life experiences

Anxiety [specify level], death

Behavior, risk-prone health body image, disturbed conflict, decisional (specify)

Coping, defensive

Coping, ineffective

Coping, readiness for enhanced

Decision making, readiness for enhanced denial, ineffective

Dignity, risk for compromised human distress, moral

Energy field, disturbed fear

Grieving

Grieving, complicated; grieving, risk for complicated; hope, readiness for enhanced

Hopelessness

Identity, disturbed personal post-trauma syndrome, post-trauma syndrome, risk for power

Readiness for enhanced powerlessness

Powerlessness, risk for rape-trauma syndrome

Relationships, readiness for enhanced

Religiosity, impaired religiosity, ready for enhanced religiosity, risk for impaired

Relocation stress syndrome

Risk for resilience

Impaired individual resilience

Readiness for enhanced resilience

Risk for compromised self-concept

Readiness for enhanced self-esteem

Chronic low self-esteem

Situational low self-esteem

Risk for situational low sorrow, chronic

Spiritual distress

Spiritual distress, risk for

Spiritual well-being, readiness for enhanced

ELIMINATION—Ability to excrete waste products

Bowel ncontinence

Constipation

Constipation, perceived

Constipation, risk for

Diarrhea

Motility, dysfunctional gastrointestinal

Motility, risk for dysfunctional gastrointestinal urinary elimination, impaired

Urinary elimination, readiness for enhanced

Urinary incontinence, functional

Urinary incontinence, overflow

Urinary incontinence, reflex

Urinary incontinence, risk for urge

Urinary incontinence, stress

Urinary incontinence, urge

Urinary retention [acute/chronic]

FOOD/FLUID—Ability to maintain intake of and utilize nutrients and liquids to meet physiological needs

Breastfeeding

Effective breastfeeding

Ineffective breastfeeding, interrupted

Dentition, impaired

Electrolyte imbalance

Risk for failure to thrive, adult

Feeding pattern, ineffective infant

Fluid balance, readiness for enhanced

Fluid volume, deficient hyper/hypotonic

Fluid volume, deficient [isotonic]

Fluid volume, excess

Fluid volume, risk for deficient

Fluid volume, risk for imbalanced glucose

Risk for unstable blood +liver function

Risk for impaired Nausea

Nutrition: less than body requirements

Imbalanced nutrition: more than body requirements

Imbalanced nutrition: risk for more than body requirements

Imbalanced nutrition, readiness for enhanced

Oral mucous membrane, impaired swallowing, impaired

HYGIENE—Ability to perform activities of daily living self-care, readiness for enhanced

Self-care deficit

Bathing self-care deficit

Dressing self-care deficit

Feeding self-care deficit

Toileting neglect, self

NEUROSENSORY—Ability to perceive, integrate, and respond to internal and external cues

Confusion

Acute confusion

Risk for acute confusion, chronic

Infant behavior, disorganized

Infant behavior, readiness for enhanced organized infant behavior, risk for disorganized

Memory, impaired neglect, unilateral

Peripheral neurovascular dysfunction, risk for

Sensory perception, disturbed (specify: visual, auditory, kinesthetic, gustatory, tactile, olfactory)

Stress overload

PAIN/DISCOMFORT—Ability to control internal/external environment to maintain comfort

Comfort, impaired

Comfort, readiness for enhanced pain, acute

Pain, chronic

RESPIRATION—Ability to provide and use oxygen to meet physiological needs

Airway clearance, ineffective

Aspiration, risk for breathing pattern

Ineffective gas exchange, impaired

Ventilation, impaired spontaneous

Ventilatory weaning response, dysfunctional

SAFETY—Ability to provide safe, growth-promoting environment

Allergy response, latex

Allergy response, risk for latex

Body temperature, risk for imbalanced contamination

Contamination, risk for

Death syndrome, risk for sudden infant environmental interpretation syndrome

Impaired falls, risk for

Health maintenance

Ineffective home maintenance

Impaired hyperthermia

Hypothermia

Immunization status, readiness for enhanced infection, risk for

Injury, risk for

Injury, risk for perioperative positioning

Jaundice, neonatal

Maternal/fetal dyad

Risk for disturbed mobility, impaired physical

Poisoning, risk for Protection

Ineffective self-mutilation self-mutilation, risk for

Skin integrity, impaired

Skin integrity, risk for impaired

Suffocation, risk for

Suicide, risk for

Surgical recovery, delayed

Thermoregulation, ineffective

Tissue integrity, impaired

Trauma, risk for

Trauma, risk for vascular

Violence, [actual/] risk for other-directed

Violence, [actual/] risk for self-directed

Wandering [specify sporadic or continual]

SEXUALITY—Ability to meet requirements/characteristics of male/female role

Childbearing process, readiness for enhanced sexual dysfunction

Sexuality pattern, ineffective

SOCIAL INTERACTION—Ability to establish and maintain relationships

Attachment, risk for impaired

Caregiver role strain

Caregiver role strain, risk for

Communication, impaired verbal

Communication, readiness for enhanced

Conflict, parental role

Coping, ineffective community

Coping, readiness for enhanced community

Coping, compromised family

Coping, disabled family

Coping, readiness for enhanced family

Family processes, dysfunctional

Family processes, interrupted

Family processes, readiness for enhanced

Loneliness, risk for

Parenting, impaired

Parenting, readiness for enhanced

Parenting, risk for impaired

Role performance, ineffective
Social Interaction, impaired
Social Isolation
TEACHING/LEARNING—Ability to incorporate and use information to achieve healthy lifestyle/optimal wellness
Development, risk for delayed growth
Risk for disproportionate growth and development
Delayed +health behavior
Risk-prone +health management
Ineffective self knowledge, deficient (specify)
Knowledge (specify)
Readiness for enhanced noncompliance
Therapeutic regimen management, ineffective
Therapeutic regimen management, ineffective family
Therapeutic regimen management, readiness for enhanced
Source: NANDA, 2011.

    < When combined with a contributing cause, an example of a nursing diagnosis of this type is

       < Self-care deficit related to bilateral forearm casts

2. Risk: This problem

    < Could develop in the future because of the presence of specific risk factors

    < Is almost inevitable unless nursing measures are implemented to stop the progression of the risk factors

    < Is validated by the presence of the risk factors

    < When combined with a contributing cause, an example of a nursing diagnosis of this type is

       < Risk for impairment of skin integrity related to inability to get out of bed without assistance

3. Possible: This problem

    < Could develop if additional risk factors develop

    < But will not develop until enough risk factors are present to change this diagnosis to a "risk" problem

   ‹ When combined with a contributing cause, an example of a nursing diagnosis of this type is

      ‹ Possible fluid volume deficit related to occasional nausea

4. Wellness: This is a progression from one level of wellness to a higher level of wellness

   ‹ Cannot be used unless the patient has indicated a desire for a greater level of wellness and

   ‹ The level of functioning on the patient's part must be already effective

   ‹ Because the client is already healthy for this diagnosis to be used, no etiology is included because there is no problem

   ‹ An example of a nursing diagnosis of this type is

      ‹ Readiness for enhanced therapeutic regimen management

5. Syndrome: This diagnosis

   ‹ Includes a group of nursing diagnoses that all relate to a specific situation

   ‹ Indicates that a serious clinical situation has developed

   ‹ Usually there is no etiology present because the use of a syndrome diagnosis

   ‹ indicates the contributing factors in the diagnosis

   ‹ An example of a nursing diagnosis of this type is

      ‹ Relocation stress syndrome

Wilkinson (2011) stressed the importance of using the process of formulating a nursing diagnosis to help the RN progress in thinking critically. This process of selecting appropriate nursing diagnoses can assist the RN in developing the skill of evaluating a patient's current situation and accurately judging the diagnoses applicable and the nursing interventions that will most effectively assist the patient. Wilkinson (2011) recommended the following questions for the nurse who is determining a nursing diagnosis:

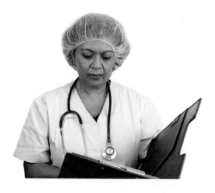

   ‹ What actual problems did I identify during assessment of the patient?

   ‹ What could be the possible causes of these problems?

   ‹ Is this patient at risk to develop other problems?

   ‹ If the patient is at risk to develop other problems, what factors are involved in making him or her subject to develop this problem?

   ‹ Did the patient express a desire to develop a higher level of wellness in his or her life?

TABLE 3-3 **Types of Nursing Problems**

Type of Problem	Description of Problem	Example of Nursing Diagnosis
Actual	This is a problem that is being experienced by the patient currently and can be validated by specific symptoms that he or she notices, along with specific signs that can observed by the nurse.	Self-care deficit related to bilateral forearm casts
Risk	This is a problem that could develop in the future because of the presence of specific risk factors. The problem is almost inevitable unless nursing measures are implemented to stop the progression of the risk factors. The presence of the risk factors validates the diagnosis.	Risk for impairment of skin integrity related to inability to get out of bed without assistance
Possible	This is a problem that could develop if additional risk factors develop. Currently, not enough risk factors are present to change this diagnosis to a "risk" problem.	Possible fluid volume deficit related to occasional nausea
Wellness	This is a progression from one level of wellness to a higher level of wellness. The patient must have indicated that there is a desire for a greater level of wellness, and the level of functioning on the patient's part must be already effective. Since the client is already healthy for this diagnosis to be utilized, no etiology is included because there is no problem.	Readiness for enhanced therapeutic regimen management
Syndrome	This diagnosis includes a group of nursing diagnoses that all relate to a specific situation. The purpose of the diagnosis is to indicate that there is a serious clinical situation that has developed. Usually there is no etiology present since the use of a syndrome diagnosis indicates the contributing factors in the diagnosis.	Relocation stress syndrome

The relationship of these questions to the process of formulating nursing diagnoses is summarized in **Figure 3-1**.

A third element can be included in the nursing diagnosis to further individual-ize it to the characteristics of the patient, that is, the signs and symptoms the RN observes in the patient. NANDA refers to the inclusion of these factors

FIGURE 3-1 **Critical Thinking Questions to Ask When Formulating Nursing Diagnoses**

What actual problems did I identify during assessment of the patient?

↓

Select actual problems of the patient
continue to review collected data.

↓

What is the severity of the actual problems of the patient?

↓

Determine if patient is a candidate for "syndrome" level of problem
continue to review collected data.

↓

What could be the possible causes of these problems?

↓

Determine etiology of actual problems
continue to review collected data.

↓

Is this patient at risk to develop other problems?

↓

Select "risk" problems of the patient
continue to review collected data.

↓

If the patient is at risk to develop other problems, what factors are involved in making him or her subject to develop this problem?

↓

Select "possible" problems of the patient
continue to review collected data.

↓

Did the patient express a desire to develop a higher level of wellness in his life?

↓

select "wellness" problems of the patient
begin initial evaluation of possible nursing actions to include in nursing plan of care
reevaluate all selected nursing diagnoses for their relevance to the patient

Source: Wilkinson, 2011.

as the "defining characteristics" of the patient's nursing diagnosis. The phrase "as evidenced by" can be included to make the diagnosis more specific to the patient's situation.

Using the nursing diagnosis of "Self-care deficit related to bilateral forearm casts" shown in Table 3-2, an example of how this could be used follows. If signs and symptoms the nurse observed that clearly indicated a self-care deficit was present were included, the diagnosis could be changed to read "Self-care deficit related to bilateral forearm casts as evidenced inability to feed self or comb hair." Such defining characteristics often are easier to add to an existing diagnosis after caring for a patient for at least an entire shift so that more lengthy observation is possible and a relationship can be established. Some experts advise using the phrase "secondary to" with a nursing diagnosis to specify the medical condition of the patient as part of the etiology (an example is "Self-care deficit related to bilateral forearm casts secondary to osteomyelitis"), but such phrasing should be used with caution, because it is all too easy to result in a medical diagnosis rather than a nursing diagnosis (Chitty & Black, 2007).

Planning

Once all applicable nursing diagnoses have been selected, the *planning* phase of the nursing process begins. In this phase the RN prioritizes the diagnoses based on the immediate needs of the patient, such as airway, breathing, and circulation. The RN collaborates with the patient to design goals to determine the choice of nursing interventions to assist the patient in resolution of the problem and also to indicate the amount of progress that is being made (Chitty & Black, 2007).

Goals are typically written to center around one of three *domains*, or categories, of learning as indicated in *Bloom's taxonomy*. Bloom was an educator who determined that learning occurred according to three basic categories of activities: *psychomotor*, *cognitive*, and *affective*. The psychomotor domain involves physical movement, and thus learning in this category can be assessed according to distance, time, and speed. The following is an example of a *nursing goal* written using this domain: "Patient will ambulate 12 feet three times daily with assistance." In comparison, the cognitive domain involves knowledge and intellectual skill. An example of a nursing goal written using this domain is "Patient will describe three signs of infection in her surgical incision by date of discharge." Finally, the affective domain involves feelings, values, and attitudes, and therefore an example of a nursing goal written using this domain is "Patient will report feeling accepting of her mastectomy surgical site by date of discharge" (Chitty & Black, 2007).

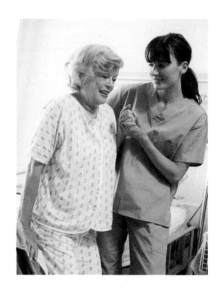

Both short-term and long-term goals should be developed, with short-term goals being achieved within hours or days and long-term goals requiring a lengthier period of time to be achieved. It is not unheard of for a long-term goal to require months to be accomplished, because it frequently can pertain to rehabilitation (Chitty & Black, 2007).

Goals can be made measurable through the development of *outcome criteria*. Outcome criteria specify the terms under which the goal will be met. Each goal can have several outcome criteria. Outcome criteria describe the conditions under which the patient will act to accomplish the goal and ultimately solve the problem and therefore are indicated by the phrase "as evidenced by" written after the goal. For example, if the goal is "Patient will report feeling accepting of her mastectomy surgical site by date of discharge," the accompanying outcome criteria would be incorporated into the goal as "Patient will report feeling accepting of her mastectomy surgical site by date of discharge as evidenced by (1) asking to view site by postoperative day 3 and (2) asking to perform dressing change without assistance by date of discharge" (Chitty & Black, 2007). If the goal and outcome criteria are written correctly, they should give a clear indication of the nursing interventions needed to assist in the accomplishment of the goals.

Intervention

Both short-term and long-term goals are written during the planning stage of the nursing process. These are particularly important because, along with the outcome criteria that make them measurable, they indicate the nursing orders that dictate the nursing interventions needed to fulfill the goals. Each goal will have its own set of nursing orders, such as "instruct on dressing change procedure prior to discharge" (Chitty & Black, 2007).

There are three basic types of nursing interventions: dependent, independent, and interdependent (**Table 3-4**). *Dependent nursing interventions* require supervision from another healthcare professional, such as a physician or a nurse practitioner. The supervision is necessary because the intervention requires an order for an action that is outside the scope of practice for the RN. For example, medication administration requires that an initial order is written by a physician or a nurse practitioner who has prescribing privileges that cover the substance being ordered.

In comparison, *independent nursing interventions* are those that require no supervision from personnel other than the RN. The nurse will have all

TABLE 3-4 Types of Nursing Interventions		
Type of Intervention	**Description**	**Example**
dependent	Requires supervision from another health-care professional, such as a physician or a nurse practitioner. The supervision is necessary because the intervention will require an order for an action that is outside the scope of practice for the registered nurse.	Administration of a medication will require an initial order to be written by a physician or nurse practitioner
independent	Requires no supervision from personnel other than the registered nurse. The nurse will have all necessary information and skill needed to implement them.	Observe the patient's urine hourly for color and clarity
interdependent	Requires collaboration and consultation with other healthcare professionals during the implementation of the action. Direct supervision from the other healthcare professional is not required because the intervention is not one that is necessarily outside of the RN's scope of practice, but consultation is required because the other professional has expertise that the RN usually does not possess.	Nursing order is written for an intervention involving a specific type of breathing exercise with which the RN is only vaguely familiar. The assistance of the facility's respiratory therapist will be required.

necessary information and skill needed to implement them. An example of an intervention could be to observe the patient's urine hourly for color and clarity. Most types of nursing interventions that involve teaching are usually independent unless they involve instruction on specific areas of expertise that are unfamiliar to the RN or are outside of his or her scope of practice (Chitty & Black, 2007).

Finally, *interdependent nursing interventions* require collaboration and consultation with other healthcare professionals during the implementation of the action. Direct supervision from another healthcare professional is not required because the intervention is not one that is necessarily outside of the RN's scope of practice, but consultation is required because the other professional has expertise the RN usually does not possess. For example, this could be required if a nursing order is written for an intervention involving a specific type of breathing exercise with which the RN is only vaguely familiar. Thus, the RN would develop an interdependent nursing intervention requiring the assistance of the facility's respiratory therapist (Chitty & Black, 2007).

As nursing orders are written and nursing interventions are developed, it is very important to remember that the interventions must be both patient-centered and related to a specific goal. This means the intervention clearly provides for individualized care for the patient based on his or her current health status in its comprehensive state, both physical and psychosocial, and also considering his or her knowledge needs (Alfaro-Lefevre, 2009).

When considering the various needs of the patient in preparation for writing nursing interventions, it may be helpful to review Maslow's Hierarchy of Needs. Maslow was a psychologist who proposed that humans are motivated by basic needs, with some of the most basic needs requiring satisfaction before some of the higher level needs can be addressed and satisfied. This means a person who lacks adequate shelter and food must have these basic needs satisfied before he or she can address the need for a stable intimate relationship (Chitty & Black, 2007). Maslow's hierarchy is described in detail in **Figure 3-2**.

FIGURE 3-2 **Maslow's Hierarchy of Needs**

SELF-ACTUALIZATION
(individual's maximum potential is realized)

↑

ESTEEM NEEDS
(self-esteem, self-respect, self-reliance)

↑

LOVE AND BELONGING NEEDS
(healthy intimacy and relationships with others)

↑

SAFETY NEEDS
(physical safety in the form of a healthy environment and psychological safety in the form of freedom from fear and anxiety)

↑

BASIC PHYSIOLOGICAL NEEDS
(air, food, water, means of sexual satisfaction) {must be satisfied initially}

Source: Chitty & Black, 2007.

Evaluation

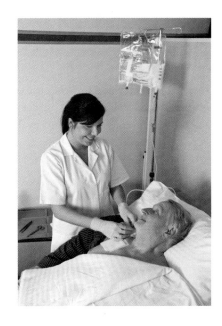

Once nursing orders have been written and nursing interventions developed and implemented, the RN can progress forward into the final stage of the nursing process. Gardner (2002) noted that it is during the *evaluation* stage when the RN decides if the goals he or she developed in collaboration with the patient were actually fulfilled. When the goals were either not fulfilled or were only partially fulfilled, the RN should gather additional data through reassessment, critically scrutinize the nursing diagnosis to determine if it is still valid, and possibly shelve it in favor of a diagnosis that is now more appropriate for the patient (Gardner, 2002). The RN can determine if goals were met by measuring the expected outcomes of the nursing interventions against the actual outcomes. Subsequently, the RN should record the outcomes as being met, unmet, or partially met (Harkreader et al., 2007). For example, if the patient goal is to experience a manageable level of discomfort as evidenced by the outcome criteria of reporting a pain level no greater than 5 on a 1- to 10-point scale and showing no signs or symptoms of discomfort such as grimacing, perspiring, and moaning, then the RN should determine if the goal was met by examining the outcome criteria. If the patient reports a level of discomfort of 4 on a 1- to 10-point scale but does demonstrate occasional grimacing, then the RN should record the goal in this case as being partially met.

When the RN determines the goal was either not met or was partially met, he or she must also determine possible reasons for the client's lack of progress toward fulfillment of the goal. Failure to achieve the goal can usually be traced to the following (Alfaro-Lefevre, 2009):

< The nursing diagnosis used to develop the goal was not accurate.
< The goal was not realistic for the patient based on his or her abilities.
< The nursing interventions were inappropriate for achieving the outcome criteria.
< The patient's medical orders changed and thus invalidated the goal.

Summary of Key Points in Chapter

The chapter described the RN's use of the nursing process in patient care. The various stages of the nursing process were reviewed: assessment, diagnosis, planning, implementation, and evaluation. The specific types of assessment were discussed, such as

- Initial assessment
- Emergency assessment
- Focused assessment
- Ongoing assessment

In addition, the mechanics of formulating nursing diagnoses as well as writing goals and outcome criteria were discussed, including

- Using the domains of learning as described in Bloom's taxonomy: affective, cognitive, and psychomotor
- Differentiating between subjective and objective data
- Formulating outcome criteria so they are measurable and specific
- Differentiating between dependent, independent, and interdependent nursing interventions
- Clearly tying the outcome criteria back to the goal

Conclusion

A primary responsibility of the RN is to create an organized plan of nursing care for the patient. The plan can only be designed within the confines of the nursing process to ensure it leads to continuity of nursing care and other health care provided in the current healthcare delivery system.

The stages of the nursing process—assessment, diagnosis, planning, implementation, and evaluation—fit together like puzzle pieces to create a plan to make inpatient care of the highest quality as well as discharge and home care follow-up priorities for the nurse and patient.

Assessment and the data collection that comprise this stage of the process are the most important parts of the entire nursing process. Part of data collection is the research needed to achieve a sufficient understanding of the patient's current health condition. We continue our data collection in the next chapter by discussing the nursing theory.

Critical Thinking Questions

1. Discuss the four types of nursing assessment and describe when it is most appropriate in your nursing practice as an RN to use each type.

   a. What type of information could you obtain using each type of nursing assessment?

   b. You are caring for Mr. Smith, a patient who was just admitted to the medical-surgical floor complaining of persistent left upper quadrant abdominal pain. Describe how you might be required to use each of the four types of nursing assessment during your care of Mr. Smith during a 12-hour shift.

2. You are the nurse manager of a nursing unit that is attempting to be more thorough in its documentation of the daily use of the nursing process. One of the personnel that you recently hired is a new graduate licensed practical nurse who is uncertain as to how the nursing process should be used in his daily patient care. Explain in simplified terms how he should be expected to use the nursing process daily.

3. In your job as a nurse manager, you find the hospital education department has just purchased some computer software that will generate nursing diagnoses based on the input of some basic information. You overhear one of the new nurses express relief that "now we have premade diagnoses, and we don't have to figure out how they can be individualized!" Explain how you would intervene to counsel this nurse on the importance of individualizing nursing diagnoses to the specific patient.

Scenarios

1. You are caring for Mr. Jones, a 52-year-old man who drove himself to the Emergency Department and presented complaining of persistent chest pain and pressure. He smokes one pack of cigarettes daily, is morbidly obese, and reports being severely stressed at his job as an accountant. His wife is a pharmaceutical representative who travels approximately 4 days per week. Together they have two teenage boys. Mr. Smith has a 28-year-old daughter from his first marriage who is married and expecting her first baby.

   Assess this situation thoroughly and try to identify all possible nursing diagnoses. When you identify a nursing diagnosis, also identify an etiology for it as well as defining characteristics, if you believe this will strengthen the diagnosis.

2. Review scenario 1. Prioritize the nursing diagnoses, select the top three, and write a goal with outcome criteria for each diagnosis. Also write at least one long-term goal.

3. Review the domains of learning that are part of Bloom's taxonomy. Use the nursing diagnoses you wrote in scenario 2 and write a goal for each diagnosis that will pertain to each domain of learning. When you finish, each diagnosis should have a goal in the psychomotor domain, a goal in the cognitive domain, and a goal in the affective domain.

4. You are caring for Mrs. Smith, a 58-year-old woman who underwent a mastectomy 3 days ago. She is scheduled to begin chemotherapy treatments for stage III breast cancer in 4 weeks. She is divorced with one 21-year-old daughter who is in college in another state. You find Mrs. Smith crying one morning when you come in to assess her at the beginning of your shift. She tells you, "I am so afraid to look at my wound. I feel so ugly!"

   a. Assess Mrs. Smith and write down all the pertinent pieces of information you identify from this scenario. Identify the information as either subjective or objective information.

   b. Try to identify all the possible nursing diagnoses that are present in scenario 4. When you identify a nursing diagnosis, also identify an etiology (primary cause) for it as well as defining characteristics.

   c. Use the nursing diagnoses that you wrote in part b and write a goal for each diagnosis that pertains to each domain of learning. When you finish, each diagnosis should have a goal in the psychomotor domain, a goal in the cognitive domain, and a goal in the affective domain.

   d. Write nursing orders and nursing interventions for each goal written in part c. Identify each nursing intervention as dependent, independent, or interdependent.

   e. Determine if the goals that you wrote in part c were met completely, partially, or not at all. If the goals were met partially or not at all, determine what could have caused this. (Because this is a fictionalized patient, be creative but realistic.)

NCLEX® Questions

Using the information you obtained from studying this chapter, go online to complete the following NCLEX®-format review questions. Visit http://go.jblearning.com/terryLPN using the access code in the front cover of your book. This interactive resource allows you to answer each question and instantly review your results. Practice until you can answer at least 75% success-fully, and then try to improve your score with each successive attempt.

1. The nursing process will help the RN (select all that apply)
   a. document the ineffectiveness of care implemented
   b. stay organized during data collection regarding the patient
   c. develop a nursing diagnosis to describe the current situation of the patient
   d. implement steps involved in the regimen of nursing care

2. When used appropriately, the nursing process will (select all that apply)
   a. require the use of critical thinking, problem-solving, and use of nursing judgment
   b. maximize errors that can occur during delivery of patient care
   c. ensure the care that is planned and implemented is individualized for the patient
   d. promote the patient's participation in his care by encouraging his autonomy

3. The type of assessment that should occur continuously throughout a patient's healthcare experience is
   a. emergency
   b. ongoing
   c. focused
   d. initial

4. The type of assessment that should include only essential data that are relevant to the patient's immediate issue is
   a. emergency
   b. ongoing
   c. focused
   d. initial

5. The type of assessment that is performed on each symptom as it is identified is
   a. emergency
   b. ongoing
   c. focused
   d. initial

6. An example of subjective data is
   a. blood pressure
   b. pulse

      c. nausea

      d. respiration

7. An example of objective data is

      a. temperature

      b. pain

      c. nausea

      d. dizziness

8. Types of problems that can be experienced by a patient include (select all that apply)

      a. actual

      b. potential

      c. wellness

      d. risk

9. The domain of Bloom's taxonomy that involves feelings, values, and attitudes is

      a. intellectual

      b. psychomotor

      c. cognitive

      d. affective

10. The domain of Bloom's taxonomy that can be assessed according to distance, time, and speed is

      a. intellectual

      b. psychomotor

      c. cognitive

      d. affective

11. "The patient will ambulate 6 feet with minimal assistance three times daily." Which domain of Bloom's taxonomy does this nursing goal fit?

      a. intellectual

      b. psychomotor

      c. cognitive

      d. affective

12. "Patient will report feeling accepting of her surgical site within 2 weeks of discharge." Which domain of Bloom's taxonomy does this nursing goal fit?

      a. intellectual

      b. psychomotor

      c. cognitive

      d. affective

13. "Patient will verbalize methods of assessing feet daily for signs and symptoms of infection." Which domain of Bloom's taxonomy does this nursing goal fit?

    a. intellectual

    b. psychomotor

    c. cognitive

    d. affective

14. The progression of Maslow's Hierarchy of Needs, from lesser to greater, is

    a. basic physiological needs, esteem needs safety needs, love and belonging needs, self-actualization

    b. basic physiological needs, love and belonging needs, safety needs, esteem needs, self-actualization

    c. basic physiological needs, self-actualization, safety needs, love and belonging needs, esteem needs

    d. basic physiological needs, safety needs, love and belonging needs, esteem needs, self-actualization

15. The RN develops a nursing diagnosis after identifying the patient has a need for self-reliance. This need falls into which section of Maslow's Hierarchy of Needs?

    a. esteem needs

    b. love and belonging needs

    c. safety needs

    d. basic physiological needs

16. The RN develops a nursing diagnosis after identifying the patient has a need for healthy intimacy. This need falls into which section of Maslow's Hierarchy of Needs?

    a. esteem needs

    b. love and belonging needs

    c. safety needs

    d. basic physiological needs

17. The RN develops a nursing diagnosis after identifying the patient has a need for self-respect. This need falls into which section of Maslow's Hierarchy of Needs?

    a. esteem needs

    b. love and belonging needs

    c. safety needs

    d. basic physiological needs

18. The RN develops a nursing diagnosis after identifying the patient has a need for adequate nutritional intake. This need falls into which section of Maslow's Hierarchy of Needs?
    a. esteem needs
    b. love and belonging needs
    c. safety needs
    d. basic physiological needs

19. The RN develops a nursing diagnosis after identifying the patient has a need for freedom from anxiety. This need falls into which section of Maslow's Hierarchy of Needs?
    a. esteem needs
    b. love and belonging needs
    c. safety needs
    d. basic physiological needs

20. The RN develops a nursing diagnosis after identifying the patient has a need for physical safety. This need falls into which section of Maslow's Hierarchy of Needs?
    a. esteem needs
    b. love and belonging needs
    c. safety needs
    d. basic physiological needs

For more information on the topics in this chapter and others, please see Appendix on p. 299 for a list of web links to additional resources.

References

Alfaro-Lefevre, R. (2009). *Applying the nursing process: A tool for critical thinking.* Philadelphia, PA: Lippincott, Williams, and Wilkins.

Chitty, K., & Black, B. (2007). *Professional nursing: Concepts and challenges* (5th ed.). Philadelphia, PA: Elsevier.

Gardner, P. (2002). *Nursing process in action.* Clifton Park, NY: Delmar.

Harkreader, H., Hogan, M., & Thobaben, M. (2007). *Fundamentals of nursing: Caring and clinical judgment* (3rd ed.). Philadelphia, PA: Elsevier.

North American Nursing Diagnosis Association (NANDA). (2011). *2009–2011 Nursing diagnoses.* Retrieved from webhome.broward.edu/~gbrickma/Forms/NANDA%25202009-2011

Quan, K. (2007). The nursing process. Retrieved from http://www.thenursing
   site.com/Articles/the%20nursing%20process.htm
Wilkinson, J. (2011). *Nursing process and critical thinking*. Philadelphia, PA:
   Prentice-Hall.

For a full suite of assignments and additional learning
activities, use the access code located in the front of
your book to visit this exclusive website: http://go.
jblearning.com/terryLPN. If you do not have an access
code, you can obtain one at the site.

www

CHAPTER OBJECTIVES

At the end of this chapter, you will be able to:

1. Discuss the major assumptions of various nursing theories.
2. Describe nursing models that are unique to specific nursing theories.
3. Select a theory of nursing that can be applied in daily nursing practice.
4. Compare and contrast the concepts of major nursing theories.

KEY TERMS

acculturation
conceptual framework
contextual stimuli
cultural awareness
cultural diversity
cultural universality
culturally congruent care
diagnostic operation
energy field
ethnicity
exploitation phase

extrapersonal stressor
focal stimuli
identification phase
interpersonal stressor
intrapersonal stressor
model
nursing theory
orientation phase
prescriptive operation
process
propositions

regulatory operation
residual stimuli
resolution phase
theory of goal attainment
theory of nursing systems
theory of self-care
theory of self-care deficit
theory of transcultural
    nursing
unitary human being

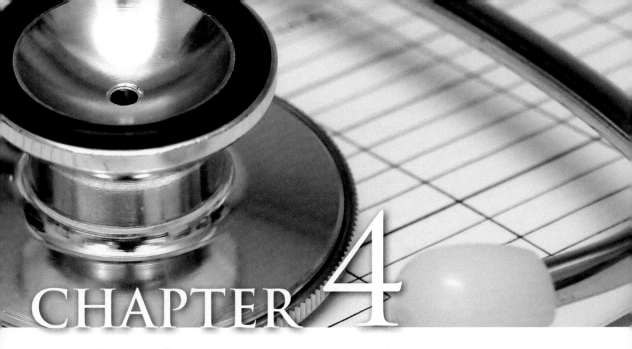

CHAPTER 4

Nursing Theory

Introduction to Nursing Theory

The nursing profession has a theoretical basis, meaning the practice of professional nursing is based on a specific body of knowledge rooted in nursing theory. *Nursing theory* refers to a group of interrelated concepts and definitions that together describe a certain view of nursing. It is that rooting of nursing practice in a theoretical basis that creates the view of nursing as a profession. Nursing theory assists the nurse in the development of critical thinking, nursing judgment, and decision making in patient care. Use of nursing theory can assist the registered nurse to (Chitty & Black, 2007)

- < Organize patient data
- < Analyze patient data
- < Understand connections between patient data
- < Determine priorities in patient data so the most important pieces of information are selected
- < Use evidence to make appropriate clinical decisions
- < Plan theoretically based nursing interventions
- < Accurately predict the outcomes of nursing interventions
- < Accurately evaluate the outcomes of nursing interventions

Nursing theories are primarily composed of processes, propositions, models, and conceptual frameworks. *Processes* are considered to be a series of actions, proposed changes, or functions that are implemented to bring about a specific result. *Propositions* are statements that explain relationships between the concepts used in a certain theory. In comparison, *models* are a documentation of the interaction that occurs between concepts and the patterns that result from that interaction. Finally, conceptual frameworks direct how these interactions occur. The *conceptual framework* defines the patient, the environment, health, and nursing, and this directs the way in which nursing care is delivered within the confines of the nursing process (Parker & Smith, 2010). Once the basic components of nursing theories are understood, the individual theories and the theorists who developed them can be studied.

Virginia Henderson's Theory of Nursing

Virginia Henderson is widely considered to be the 20th-century equivalent of Florence Nightingale. Her work as a nursing philosopher emerged at a time when there was a great need to determine the confines of nursing as a profession. She believed the definition of nursing could not be separated from the function of nursing, which she saw as assisting the person, whether ill or physically well, in performing the usual activities that contributed to his or her health or, if necessary, a peaceful death that he or she would perform without assistance if possible. Henderson believed the nurse was uniquely equipped to be a substitute for the patient, a helper to him or her, or a partner with the patient (Chitty & Black, 2007).

As part of her theory, Henderson emphasized the need to increase the patient's independence apart from the nurse so that after hospitalization, progress toward recovery would continue. In addition, the theory assumed that patients have an intrinsic desire to return to a state of health. Also, there was an assumption that nurses possessed both a willingness to serve the patient in the resumption of health and a willingness to devote themselves to the process around the clock, if the need presented itself (Parker & Smith, 2010).

Henderson believed 14 basic needs of the individual formed the basis for care delivered by the nurse. These needs formed a holistic view of the patient and also provided a multifaceted definition of the function of the nurse: to assist the patient who could not perform each of the 14 functions independently. Henderson described the 14 functions as

< Breathing
< Eating and drinking
< Elimination
< Mobility
< Sleeping/resting
< Dressing suitably for environmental temperature
< Maintaining body temperature
< Keeping body clean/grooming
< Avoiding endangering self or others in the environment
< Expressing thoughts and emotions
< Worshipping according to choice
< Receiving a sense of accomplishment from work
< Participating in recreational activities
< Learning about health and using available health facilities (Chitty & Black, 2007)

Virginia Henderson's theory of nursing included four primary concepts: the individual, the environment, health, and nursing. She saw the individual as

< Having basic needs that are all components of health
< Requiring assistance in the restoration of health
< Having an interrelationship between mind and body
< Being neither a client nor a consumer
< Being multifaceted, with physical, psychological, sociological, and spiritual needs

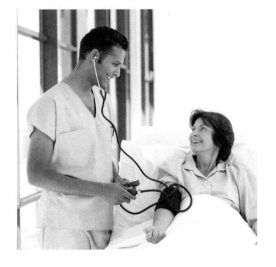

The environment of the individual was seen as the settings in which the person learns a pattern to be used for his or her day-to-day life as well as everything that affects the life of the person and his or her development. Henderson viewed health as the individual's ability to function without assistance and believed that nurses should actively engage in health promotion as well as disease prevention and the elimination of illness. Finally, she believed nursing provided a temporary assistance to the individual until he or she could return to independence (Parker & Smith, 2010). **Table 4-1** shows the basic concepts of Henderson's nursing theory.

TABLE 4-1 Basic Concepts of Virginia Henderson's Theory of Nursing	
Henderson's Concept	**Description**
individual	The individual has basic needs that are all components of health
	The individual requires assistance in the restoration of health
	The individual has an interrelationship between mind and body
	The individual is neither a client nor a consumer
	The individual is multi-faceted, with physical, psychological, sociological, and spiritual needs
environment	The environment consists of the settings in which the person learns a pattern that will be used for his day-to-day life
	The environment consists of everything that affects the life of the person and his development
health	Health is the individual's ability to function without assistance
nursing	Nursing provides a temporary assistance to the individual until he or she can return to independence
	The nurse should actively engage in health promotion, disease prevention and the elimination of illness
Source: Parker & Smith, 2010.	

Imogene King's Theory of Nursing

Imogene King is significant to nursing theory because of her *theory of goal attainment*. She proposed that nursing is a process by which the nurse and the client interact to develop a perception of each other and the client's situation and, as a result, develop goals for the client and collaborate on a means to achieve those goals. King consistently referred to the patient in her theory as "the client" (McElwen & Wills, 2010).

King's theory proposed that the nurse's focus was on issues of importance to the client; this focus was such a priority it was likely to prevent mutual goal setting from occurring. King believed each individual had multiple interpersonal relationships as well as three interacting systems, which she labeled as personal, interpersonal, and social. These interacting systems together formed a framework that allowed the individual client to be seen in their entirety (Chitty & Black, 2007):

< The personal system provided an understanding of the client, both personally and within him- or herself.
< The interpersonal system provided an understanding of the interaction and transactions that can occur between multiple persons.
< The social system provided an understanding of social contacts with individuals in settings such as the workplace or school.

Whereas the previously mentioned theory of Virginia Henderson focused on the needs of the patient, King's theory focused on goal attainment both for the client and by the client. King believed nursing care for the client was guided by the personal, interpersonal, and social systems. The client's personal system caused the registered nurse to observe the client's perceptions, the interpersonal system caused the nurse to observe the client's multiple roles in his or her life as well as the stressors he or she experienced while interacting in each role, and the social system caused the nurse to note influences on the client's decision-making capabilities. King found interaction with the client to be of particular importance in the goal attainment theory and believed that specific steps in the communication process occurred as the client moved from a first encounter with the nurse until the desired goal was achieved. Identified as progressing in difficulty, the steps were labeled as

< Perception
< Judgment
< Action
< Reaction
< Interaction
< Transaction

King also believed that progressive difficulty of the steps required an increasing level of involvement between the nurse and the client so the nurse achieved a comprehensive understanding of the goals of the client to appropriately plan and provide nursing care. This underscored the importance of goals being set on a collaborative basis between nurse and client (Chitty & Black, 2007).

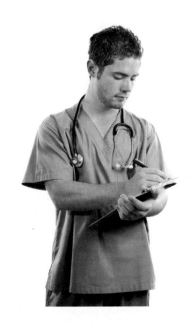

King's theory of goal attainment viewed the nursing process as consisting of four stages: assessment, planning, implementation, and evaluation. In the assessment stage, the perceptions of the nurse and client are developed, mutual communication occurs, and interaction develops. In the planning stage, decisions are made about goals, and there is mutual agreement regarding the means used to attain those goals. During the implementation stage, transactions are made, and the subsequent evaluation stage determined if the goal was attained; if attainment did not occur, an investigation ensued to discover the reason (Alligood & Tomey, 2006).

Several primary concepts are considered to be intrinsic to King's theory:

- Nursing's goal is to help the client maintain his or her health so the individual can function in his or her role; nursing is an interpersonal process that is influenced by both the nurse and the client's perceptions. Nursing is a process that consists of action, reaction, interaction, and transaction.
- The individual is made up of an open system that is in transaction with the environment, meaning the client cannot be separated from his or her environment; the individual has a spiritual component, can think, use language, make choices, and choose from several courses of action; each individual is different in his or her wants, needs, and goals, is unique, holistic, of worth, able to think rationally, and participate in decision making in most instances.
- Health is considered to be a dynamic state in the individual's life cycle; thus, illness is considered to be an incident that interferes with the smooth progression of that life cycle.
- Environment for the client is constantly changing, and the individual constantly interacts with his or her environment to maintain a state of health; it is the interaction with the environment that influences each individual's adjustments to his or her life and state of health (Tomey & Alligood, 2006).

Table 4-2 summarizes the basic concepts of King's theory.

Madeleine Leininger's Theory of Nursing

Madeleine Leininger's primary contribution to theoretical nursing was the theory of nursing known as *transcultural nursing*. She based her ideas on principles unique to the science of anthropology. After recognizing the world was rapidly becoming one in which humans would have to function multiculturally, she proposed that nursing was failing to provide nurses with adequate cultural knowledge. Leininger believed that culture is learned, passed from

TABLE 4-2 Basic Concepts of Imogene King's Theory of Nursing	
Concept	**Description**
nursing	Nursing has as its goal to help the client maintain health so that the individual can function in his or her role. Nursing is an interpersonal process that is influenced by perceptions of both the nurse and the client. Nursing is a process that consists of action, reaction, interaction, and transaction.
individual	The individual is made up of an open system that is in transaction with the environment. The client cannot be separated from his or her environment. The individual has a spiritual component, can think, use language, make choices, and choose from several courses of action. Each individual is different in wants, needs, and goals, is unique, holistic, of worth, able to think rationally, and participate in decision making.
health	Health is a dynamic state in the individual's life cycle. Illness is an incident that interferes with the smooth progression of that life cycle.
environment	Environment for the client is constantly changing, and the individual constantly interacts with his or her environment to maintain a state of health. It is the interaction with the environment that influences each individual's adjustments to his life and his state of health.

Source: Tomey & Alligood, 2006.

one generation to the next, and can be observed in a person's actions, words, behavioral rules, and symbols (Alligood & Tomey, 2006).

A primary concept in the theory of transcultural nursing is that of *cultural diversity*, which are the variations observed between cultures. The nurse who is capable of recognizing the variations among cultures can avoid inadvertently stereotyping patients and thus assuming that all patients will respond to a "generic" plan for nursing care in the same manner. Similarly, another important concept of the theory is that of *cultural universality*, meaning the similarities that exist in various cultures when they are scrutinized. The nurse who recognizes such similarities is capable of recognizing the impact that health, healthy practices, and instruction on the maintenance of wellness have on the general well-being of entire cultural groups (Alligood & Tomey, 2006).

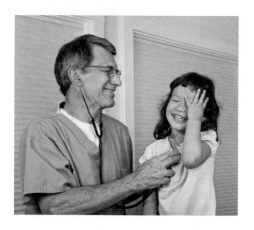

The goal of the theory of transcultural nursing is to plan culturally congruent nursing care based on knowledge that has been culturally defined. Leininger encouraged the registered nurse to be creative in attempts to discover the cultural aspects of the needs of patients and then use these discoveries in designing culturally congruent nursing care. She believed caring was the essence of nursing, and such caring encompassed nursing practice that respects the patient's culture. When culturally congruent care is implemented appropriately, the outcome will be a high level of health and well-being for the patient (Chitty & Black, 2007).

Several concepts are considered to be unique to Leininger's theory:

< *Ethnicity* is the awareness of belonging to a specific group.
< *Acculturation* means members of a minority group usually assume the beliefs, practices, and values of the dominant cultural group in the society so that a blending of the cultural group occurs.
< *Cultural awareness* occurs when the nurse examines his or her own background to assist in recognizing the existence of biases, prejudices, and assumptions that are present about other people.
< *Culturally congruent care* is nursing care that respects the patient's values and life patterns (McElwen & Wills, 2010).

Table 4-3 highlights the concepts that are unique to Leininger's theory of nursing.

TABLE 4-3 Concepts Unique to Leininger's Theory

Concept	Description
ethnicity	Awareness of belonging to a specific group
acculturation	Members of a minority group assume beliefs, practices, and values of the dominant cultural group so that a blending of the cultural group occurs
cultural awareness	Nurse examines his own background to assist in recognizing existence of biases, prejudices, and assumptions
cultural congruent care	Nursing care respects patient's values and life patterns

Source: McElwen & Wills, 2010.

Betty Neuman's Theory of Nursing

Betty Neuman's theory of nursing is a system theory that has its roots in stress theory and the mental health community. Neuman proposed that each person is a system, meaning a group of characteristics and factors contained within a specific range of responses that may occur, and these factors and responses are in turn housed within a basic structure. Each person (usually referred to as a client in Neuman's theory) has developed a range of responses to the environment that is considered to be normal for his or her system. A deviation from the client's usual state of health is noted by determining the responses to the environment are no longer capable of protecting him or her from stressors. Within each client are a set of internal resistance factors that seek to stabilize him or her as a system and return that person to his or her usual state of wellness. The client as a system is in a state of homeostasis when there is a constant and ever-changing process of input, output, feedback, and subsequent compensation in response (McElwen & Wills, 2010).

Neuman's theory of nursing has specific concepts that are unique to it (**Table 4-4**):

- Human being: Consists of a client system with multiple layers. Each layer is composed of five subsystems:
  - Physiological
  - Psychological
  - Sociocultural
  - Spiritual
  - Developmental
- Environment: The total internal and external forces that interact with a client. The internal environment is within the client, whereas the external environment is outside the client.
- Health: Seen as being synonymous with wellness.
- Nursing: Viewed as being concerned with all variables that affect the client's response to a stressor (McElwen & Wills, 2010).

Neuman's theory of nursing focuses in large part on stressors that can influence the stability of the client system. Such stressors can be classified as intrapersonal, interpersonal, or extrapersonal. *Intrapersonal stressors* are the internal stressors that occur within the boundaries of the client's system, such as various disease processes. *Interpersonal stressors* are those that occur in the external environment outside of the client system but close to the system boundaries. This could include the client's multiple roles in his or her family and relationships with friends. Finally, *extrapersonal stressors* occur in the external environment outside of the client system but farther away from the system boundaries. This could include the client's employment status as well as various resources available to the client in the community (Alligood & Tomey, 2006).

TABLE 4-4 Concepts Unique to Neuman's Theory of Nursing

Concept	Description	Example
Human being	Consists of a client system with multiple layers; each layer is composed of five subsystems: a. physiological b. psychological c. sociocultural d. spiritual, and e. developmental	
Environment	The total internal and external forces that interact with a client	The internal environment is within the client; the external environment is outside the client.
Health	Synonymous with wellness	
Nursing	Concerned with all of the variables that affect the client's response to a stressor	
Intrapersonal stressors	Internal stressors that occur within the boundaries of the client's system	Various disease processes
Interpersonal stressors	Those that occur in the external environment outside of the client system but close to the system boundaries	This could include client's multiple roles in his family and relationships with friends.
Extrapersonal stressors	Those that occur in the external environment outside of the client system but farther away from the system boundaries	This could include client's employment status as well as various resources available to the client in the community.

Source: McElwen & Wills, 2010; Alligood & Tomey, 2006.

Florence Nightingale's Theory of Nursing

Florence Nightingale is considered to be the first nursing theorist, proposing the following (McKenna, 2002):

< Nursing requires a spiritual "calling" to be practiced effectively.
< Nursing requires specific educational requirements and specific training to be implemented appropriately.
< Nursing is not synonymous with the practice of medicine.
< Nursing is both an art and a science.
< Nursing is most effectively practiced through altering the environment to produce optimal conditions for the patient.

Nightingale had high expectations for nurses even in the 19th century. She indicated in her writings that the nurse should closely observe the patient to note changes and accurately make judgments about the patient's condition. She proposed that nursing education should be a combination of both clinical and classroom instruction. Nightingale believed that because nursing required a spiritual calling, the nurse should be equipped to assist the patient who was experiencing spiritual distress through some level of health teaching and ultimately health promotion (Alligood & Tomey, 2006).

A significant part of Nightingale's theory was the belief that a patient's health was a direct result of his or her environment. She recognized how providing for clean air and water, sanitation, light, and bathing could contribute to a patient's recovery from significant illness. She addressed the nurse's responsibility to not only feed the patient but to also document the amount of food eaten and the patient's response to the diet served. Nightingale also proposed that excessive noise in hospitals should be addressed because of the importance of adequate rest to the recovering patient (Chitty & Black, 2007).

Specific assumptions are unique to Nightingale's theory of nursing but also form the basis for nursing theories that were developed in later years (**Table 4-5**):

< Nursing: Nightingale believed the trained nurse used scientific principles in his or her work, applied skill in observing patients' health and both reporting and documenting changes in the health status, and intervened as necessary to facilitate the recovery of the patient.
< Person: Nightingale usually spoke of the individual as the patient. Although the nurse was believed to have the primary control regarding

TABLE 4-5 Basic Concepts of Nightingale's Theory of Nursing

Concept	Description
nursing	The trained nurse uses scientific principles, applies skill in observing patients' health and both reporting and documenting changes in health status, and intervenes as necessary in order to facilitate recovery. ‹ Nursing requires a spiritual "calling" ‹ Nursing requires specific educational requirements and specific training ‹ Nursing is not synonymous with medicine ‹ Nursing is both an art and a science, and ‹ Nursing is involves altering the environment for optimal conditions
person	Health equates with being "well" and with using every available resource to make certain that a person lives his life to greatest extent possible. Both disease and illness can benefit the person by repairing damage that occurred when he or she did not address health problems.
health	Although the nurse was believed to have primary control regarding the patient's recovery since she was responsible for performing tasks and arranging the environment to speed the recovery process, the patient was seen as an individual.
environment	The environment is everything outside of the person that can affect both the ill person and the well individual. Nightingale wrote about the need for improved sanitary living conditions and hygiene, health problems that unsanitary conditions could cause, and ways to remedy them.

Source: Tomey & Alligood, 2006.

the patient's recovery because she was responsible for performing tasks for the patient and arranging the environment in such a way as to speed the recovery process, the patient was seen as an individual. Nightingale instructed nurses to ask patients about their preferences, for instance, regarding meal times, to give the patient some small measure of control regarding his or her surroundings.

‹ Health: Nightingale viewed health as being "well" and as using every available resource to make certain a person lived life to the greatest extent possible. She believed that both disease and illness could benefit the person by repairing damage that occurred when he or she did not address health problems. To maintain the health of the individual, she believed that control of the environment on the part of the nurse as well as social responsibility was necessary.

< Environment: Nightingale viewed the environment as everything outside of the person that could affect the person both with an illness and without. She believed the poor of her day, who frequently lived in the most desperate of conditions, could benefit greatly from changes in their environments that would not only affect their bodies but also influence their minds. Nightingale essentially designed rural health care and wrote exhaustively on the need for improved sanitary living conditions and hygiene, the health problems that unsanitary conditions could cause, and ways to remedy such situations (Tomey & Alligood, 2006).

Dorothea Orem's Theory of Nursing

Dorothea Orem was a nursing theorist who was a proponent of individuals being self-reliant and responsible for the health care of themselves and their family members. Orem actually designed three theories that involved self-care, self-care deficit, and the nursing system that fit together to form a larger theory known as the self-care deficit theory (Alligood & Tomey, 2006). The *theory of self-care* described why individuals choose to care for themselves and how they implement the care. The *theory of self-care deficit* explained why individuals can be helped through nursing and also described how such care can be beneficial. The *theory of nursing systems* proposed relationships that must be both developed and maintained in order for nursing to be implemented and attempted to explain the nature of these relationships (Tomey & Alligood, 2006).

Orem's theory of nursing focused on the capacity of the patient to provide self-care and the process of developing nursing interventions to fulfill the individual's unmet needs for self-care. The theory proposed that the patient has a self-care deficit consisting of the degree to which he or she is unable to provide self-care. Because of this self-care deficit the nurse will need to regulate the nursing system, which consists of various relationships. Therefore, an overriding assumption of the theory is that the ordinary individual in modern society has a need to be in control of his or her own life (Chitty & Black, 2007).

Orem further proposed that the nurse should develop appropriate care for the individual through three different types of operations: diagnostic, prescriptive, or regulatory. A *diagnostic operation* establishes the nurse–patient relationship and determines the individual's ability to provide self-care. The

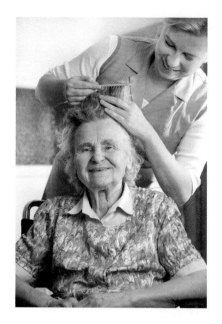

patient's ability to provide effective self-care will be assessed by the nurse to determine a baseline and measure the extent to which the patient has a limitation in providing his or her own self-care. These limitations are documented as self-care deficits. In comparison, ***prescriptive operations*** are used in a planning stage when the nurse confirms with the patient that the baseline assessment is accurate and a plan of care is developed. Finally, in ***regulatory operations*** the nurse designs and generates a system for nursing care for the patient that can range from completely compensatory, providing the highest level of care for the patient with little if any ability to provide self-care, to only supportive or educational, providing assistance to the individual who has the ability to provide self-care but needs additional knowledge (Chitty & Black, 2007).

Some major assumptions are unique to Orem's theory of nursing (**Table 4-6**):

< Nursing is considered to be an art, a helping service, and a technology; the goal of nursing is to assist the individual in becoming capable of meeting his or her own self-care needs.
< Health is considered to be both structural and functional soundness; includes every quality that makes a person human.

TABLE 4-6 Basic Concepts of Orem's Theory of Nursing

Concept	Description
nursing	Considered to be an art as well as a helping service, as well as a technology; the goal of nursing is to assist the individual in becoming capable of meeting his own self-care needs
health	Considered to be both structural and functional soundness; includes every quality that makes a person human
human being	Considered to be a being with universal as well as developmental needs and being capable of self-care on a continuous basis
nursing problem	Occurs when there is a deficit in a universal, developmental, or health-derived/health-related condition

Source: Chinn & Kramer, 2010.

‹ Human being is considered to have universal and developmental needs and to be capable of self-care on a continuous basis.

‹ Nursing problem occurs when there is a deficit in a universal, developmental, or health-derived/health-related condition (Chinn & Kramer, 2010).

Ida Orlando's Theory of Nursing

Ida Orlando was one of the first nursing theorists to write extensively about the nursing process and the nurse–patient relationship. She believed the role of the nurse was to assess and ultimately meet the patient's immediate need for assistance. She believed the patient's presenting behavior was indirectly a call for assistance, although the help needed from the nurse might actually be different from that originally anticipated. Because of this it is the responsibility of the nurse to explore with patients the meaning of their behavior. This can best be done by using the nurse's perception about the patient's behavior, thoughts about the perception, or feelings derived from those thoughts.

There are four primary dimensions to Orlando's theory of nursing (Chinn & Kramer, 2010):

‹ Distress: Experienced by the patient who has unmet needs.

‹ Nursing role: To assess the patient's unmet needs and meet his or her immediate need for assistance. The nurse should recognize the patient's behavior may not, in fact, represent the true need that is occurring; thus, the nurse should validate her or her understanding of the unmet need with the patient.

‹ Nursing actions: Designed to directly or indirectly provide for the patient's immediate needs.

‹ Outcome: Change in the behavior of the patient indicating either a relief from immediate distress or an unmet need; can be noted both through verbal and nonverbal communication with the patient.

Apart from these four dimensions, other concepts unique to Orlando's theory (Chinn & Kramer, 2010):

‹ Nursing: Viewed as being responsive to the individual who is experiencing a sense of helplessness or is anticipating that such helplessness will occur

‹ Health: Seen as a sense of well-being and comfort, with needs being fulfilled

< Human being: Considered to be a developmental being with needs
< Nursing client: Person under medical care who either cannot fulfill his or her medical needs or cannot carry out medical treatment without assistance from the nurse
< Nursing problem: Distress experienced by the nursing client; the distress may be caused by physical limitation, adverse reactions to the nursing client's environment, or experiences that can prevent the person from being able to make others aware of his or her needs
< Nursing process: An interaction of the patient's behavior, the nurse's reaction to that behavior, and nursing actions that are chosen for the benefit of the nursing client

Orlando's theory focused to the greatest degree on understanding problematic situations in which the nurse recognizes the patient is demonstrating behavior that is a cue for assistance. The patient's behavior will in turn generate a response from the nurse, a unique reaction that consists of the nurse's perceptions, feelings evoked, and the nurse's past experiences and acquired knowledge. The nurse and the patient will need to communicate to determine the meaning of the patient's behavior and the help required. Once the patient's situation has been made clear, it will no longer be considered problematic; once the patient's most pressing needs have been identified and resolved, the patient's situation will improve and a new equilibrium will develop (Alligood & Tomey, 2006).

Regarding the significance of Orlando's theory, Chitty & Black (2007) noted that it is very useful as a theory to be implemented in practice. It specifies how nursing clients can be involved in the decision-making process of the nurse and can guide interactions to yield predictable outcomes. Nurses can use the theory as they individualize care for each patient. This can be done by paying attention to the nursing client's behavior, carefully verifying ideas that the nurse derives from interaction with the client, and identifying client needs that appear to be of most concern to the individual (Chitty & Black, 2007). **Table 4-7** summarizes the basic concepts of Orlando's theory.

Hildegard Peplau's Theory of Nursing

Hildegard Peplau made great strides in promoting nursing professionalism through the use of credentialing as well as advanced practice nursing. However, her theory of nursing is remarkable on its own because of its contribution

TABLE 4-7 Basic Concepts of Orlando's Theory of Nursing

Concept	Description
distress	Experienced by the patient who has unmet needs
nursing role	To assess the patient's unmet needs and meet his or her immediate need for assistance; the nurse should recognize that the patient's behavior may not represent the true need that is occurring, thus, the nurse should validate her or her understanding of the unmet need with the patient
nursing actions	Designed to provide for the patient's immediate needs
outcome	Change in the behavior of the patient indicating either a relief from immediate distress or an unmet need
nursing	Viewed as being responsive to the individual who is experiencing a sense of helplessness
health	Seen as being a sense of well being and comfort, with needs being fulfilled
human being	Considered to be a developmental being with needs
nursing client	Person under medical care who either cannot fulfill his medical needs or cannot carry out medical treatment without assistance from the nurse
nursing problem	Distress experienced by the nursing client; may be caused by physical limitation, adverse reactions to the nursing client's environment, or experiences that can prevent the person from being able to make others aware of his or her needs
nursing process	An interaction of the patient's behavior, the nurse's reaction to that behavior, and nursing actions that are chosen for the benefit of the nursing client

Source: Chinn & Kramer, 2010.

to the study of psychiatric nursing. Peplau identified the nurse–patient relationship as consisting of four phases: orientation, identification, exploitation, and resolution (Tomey & Alligood, 2006). In the ***orientation phase*** the client meets the nurse for the first time, with both being strangers. In this phase the problem is defined and the type of service required by the patient is specified. The client will seek assistance, communicate his or her needs, ask questions, discuss his or her preconceptions, and also share past experiences (Chinn & Kramer, 2010).

The ***identification phase*** of the nurse–patient relationship involves interdependent goal setting by the nurse and patient so the ***exploitation phase***

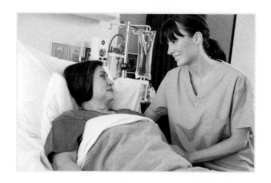

can use professional resources to assist in designing problem-solving alternatives. This enables the individual to feel a part of the helping environment. As the relationship progresses into the *resolution phase*, the professional relationship with the nurse is terminated once the patient's needs have been met through collaboration between the nurse and the patient (Chinn & Kramer, 2010).

Peplau proposed that, during the course of the nurse–patient relationship, six different nursing roles can be assumed: stranger, resource person, teacher, leader, surrogate, and counselor. The nurse's time spent in these roles varies depending on the work setting (Tomey & Alligood, 2006). During the course of the nurse–patient relationship, the roles progresses as follows (Chinn & Kramer, 2010):

< Stranger: The nurse and the patient meet initially; the nurse is careful to generate an accepting trust-building environment.
< Teacher: The nurse supplies knowledge for the patient in response to a need that has been identified or an interest the patient has communicated.
< Resource person: The nurse supplies specific information for the patient in response to a new problem that has been revealed or a new situation that has occurred.
< Counselor: Helps the patient understand and incorporate the meaning of the patient's current life situation; provides guidance as needed and encourages the patient to make changes as needed.
< Surrogate: Acts on the patient's behalf as an advocate.
< Leader: Assists the patient to assume the maximum responsibility for meeting his or her treatment goals in a way that satisfied the collaboratively set goals of the patient and the nurse.

Peplau's theory of interpersonal relations focused on the nurse–patient relationship rather than spotlighting the patient alone, with nursing care seen as occurring within the boundaries of the nurse–patient relationship (**Table 4-8**). The therapeutic interpersonal relationship was viewed as having two goals (Chitty & Black, 2007):

< Survival of the patient
< Patient's understanding of his or her health problems, learning from the problems as new behavior patterns began to develop.

FIGURE 4-8 Peplau's Nurse's Roles in the Nurse–Patient Relationship

Role	Description	Example
stranger	The nurse and the patient meet initially; the nurse is careful to generate an accepting environment that is trust-building.	The nurse and patient meet initially, having previously been strangers to each other.
teacher	The nurse supplies knowledge for the patient in response to a need that has been identified or an interest that the patient has communicated.	The patient communicated that colon cancer runs in his family and he would like to learn how to incorporate additional fiber into his daily diet.
resource person	The nurse supplies specific information for the patient in response to a new problem that has been revealed or a new situation that has occurred.	The patient communicates that she has been experiencing menstrual cycles that are heavier than usual.
counselor	Counselor-helps the patient understand and incorporate the meaning of the patient's current life situation; provides guidance as needed and encourages the patient to make changes as needed.	The patient communicates that he has just been diagnosed with lung cancer.
surrogate	Surrogate-acts on the patient's behalf as an advocate.	At the patient's request, the nurse discusses a situation with the patient's family member that the patient cannot yet address.
leader	Leader-assists the patient to assume the maximum responsibility for meeting his or her treatment goals in a way that satisfies the collaboratively set goals of the patient and the nurse.	The nurse contracts with the patient for him to complete all of the sessions of outpatient therapy and lets it be the patient's responsibility to arrange for transportation to and from the clinic.

Source: Theory of Interpersonal Relations, n.d.

Martha Rogers' Theory of Nursing

Rogers' theory of unitary human beings can be a difficult one for the registered nurse to grasp because of its complexity. Rogers was greatly influenced by the theory of relativity of Einstein, and her work also can be compared with von Bertalanffy's general system theory (Tomey & Alligood, 2006). Rogers' theory is particularly important because of its emphasis on nursing as both an art and a science (**Table 4-9**).

TABLE 4-9 Basic Concepts Unique to Rogers's Theory of Nursing

Concept	Description
unitary human being	An integration of the human being and his or her environment Human beings are one with the universe The unitary human being cannot be separated from his or her environment
nursing	Purpose is to both identify and examine the unitary human being Nursing should support the patient as he progresses through life and subsequently achieves maximum potential for health
energy field	Basic unit of both the living and nonliving entities in the universe Energy fields vary constantly in intensity, density, and extent There were no boundaries that prevent energy from flowing between energy fields Human energy and the environmental field are involved in a constant exchange of energy
health	Defined by the patient The nurse should assist the patient in moving toward his definition of health
scope of nursing	Scope of nursing should include: maintenance of health promotion of health prevention of disease formulation of nursing diagnosis development of nursing intervention, and actions for rehabilitation

Source: Tomey & Alligood, 2006; Reed & Shearer, 2011.

Rogers' viewed nursing as being synonymous with a body of knowledge and as a learned profession that must be based on scientific evidence. Such scientific knowledge should be used to improve the day-to-day existence of the *unitary human being*, which Rogers defined as being an integration of the human being and his or her environment (Tomey & Alligood, 2006).

Rogers' definition of the unitary human being is a complex one, because Rogers described the human being and the environment as energy fields greater than the sum of their parts. The concept is that nursing has as its purpose to both identify and examine the unitary human being. Rogers believed that nursing should support the patient as he or she progresses through life and subsequently achieves maximum potential for health. The patient defines for himself or herself what health means, and therefore the nurse should assist the patient in moving toward that goal. She saw the scope of nursing as consisting of (Tomey & Alligood, 2006)

< Maintenance of health
< Promotion of health
< Prevention of disease
< Formulation of nursing diagnosis
< Development of nursing intervention
< Actions for rehabilitation

Some of Rogers' most complex ideas centered around the "unitary human being." She believed human beings are one with the universe, and subsequently the unitary human being cannot be separated from his or her environment. She further proposed a basic unit of both living and nonliving entities in the universe, which she referred to as the *energy field*, and these energy fields were constantly varying in intensity, density, and extent. She believed there were no boundaries to prevent energy from flowing between energy fields, and the human energy and the environmental field were involved in a constant exchange of energy (Reed & Shearer, 2011).

Despite its complexity, Rogers' theory has relevance for the modern healthcare delivery system because of its emphasis on the inability to separate the patient's experience from his or her very existence as a human being. This is important in 21st-century healthcare where the emphasis is more on the overall continuum of care and much less on periodic episodes of ill and treatment. Her theory's emphasis on nursing based on scientific knowledge that can subsequently guide nursing practice can be argued as the forerunner of the modern emphasis on evidence-based nursing practice (Tomey & Alligood, 2006).

Sister Callista Roy's Theory of Nursing

Sister Callista Roy's theory of nursing is based on adaptation and human adaptive behavior. Roy is currently a member of the order of Sisters of Saint Joseph of Carondelet, and her theory shows that influence in her focus on the human being as a biopsychosocial system that is constantly trying to cope with the demands placed by environmental stimuli. Roy proposed that when the individual can adapt effectively to the demands of environmental stimuli, the person can maintain integrity, conserve his or her energy, and ultimately promote his or her own survival, growth, and reproduction as a human system. Recognizing this, the registered nurse will assess the patient's adaptive behavior, develop nursing diagnoses to guide development of goals and nursing interventions to promote adaptation, and ultimately modify the environment to facilitate adaptation of the patient (Chitty & Black, 2007).

Roy believed the patient is constantly interacting with an environment that is also constantly changing. To cope with the constant change in the environment, the person must use both inborn mechanisms of coping and acquired mechanisms; such mechanisms may be biological, psychological, or social in nature. The person's adaptation to environmental change is directly related to the stimulus to which he or she is exposed and adaptation level. The adaptation level consists of a zone that indicates a range of stimuli that will produce a positive response in the individual. In turn, four modes of adaptation can be used by the individual: physiological needs, self-concept, role function, and interdependence (Reed & Shearer, 2011) (**Table 4-10**).

Roy's theory departs from other theoretical proposals of nursing in her stages of the nursing process. She proposed six stages (Tomey & Alligood, 2006):

< Assess behaviors produced from the four adaptive modes.
< Assess the stimuli for the behaviors that are produced and determine if they are focal, contextual, or residual. *Focal stimuli* immediately confront the patient, *contextual stimuli* are all other stimuli present that contribute to the effect of the focal stimuli, and *residual stimuli* are environmental factors that have effects not determined in a specific situation.
< Determine a nursing diagnosis reflective of the person's current adaptive state.
< Set goals to promote the process of adaptation.
< Implement interventions that manage the stimuli and subsequently promote adaptation.

TABLE 4-10 Concepts Unique to Roy's Theory of Nursing

Concept	Description
stages of the nursing process	1. Assess behaviors produced from the four adaptive modes 2. Assess the stimuli for the behaviors that are produced and determine if they are focal, contextual, or residual; focal stimuli are those that immediately confront the patient; contextual stimuli are all other stimuli present that will contribute to the effect of the focal stimuli; and residual stimuli are environmental factors that have effects that have not been determined in a specific situational adaptation 3. Determine a nursing diagnosis reflective of the person's current adaptive state 4. Set goals to promote the process of adaptation 5. Implement interventions that will manage the stimuli and subsequently promote 6. Evaluate if adaptive goals have been met through manipulation of stimuli rather than through manipulation of the patient
adaptation	Considered to be the goal of nursing
person	Functions as an adaptive system; biopsychosocial being who is constantly interacting with the changing environment
environment	Synonymous with stimuli, focal, contextual, or residual
health	Considered to be the outcome of adaptation
nursing	Promotes both health and adaptation

< Evaluate if adaptive goals have been met through manipulation of stimuli rather than through manipulation of the patient.

Specific concepts are considered to be unique to Roy's theory (Reed & Shearer, 2011):

< Adaptation: Considered to be the goal of nursing
< Person: Functions as an adaptive system; biopsychosocial being who is constantly
< interacting with the changing environment
< Environment: Synonymous with stimuli, focal, contextual, or residual

‹ Health: Considered to be the outcome of adaptation
‹ Nursing: Promotes both health and adaptation.

Summary of Key Points in Chapter

Some of the most influential nursing theorists' contributions to nursing were discussed in this chapter, with each theorist's major assumptions, unique concepts, and developed proposals described. The following theorists were discussed:

‹ Virginia Henderson
‹ Imogene King
‹ Madeleine Leininger
‹ Betty Neuman
‹ Florence Nightingale
‹ Dorothea Orem
‹ Ida Jean Orlando
‹ Hildegard Peplau
‹ Martha Rogers
‹ Sister Callista Roy

Tables that outlined the key points developed by each theorist were included for each theory.

Conclusion

The registered nurse will develop a more in-depth understanding of the theorists and their contribution to nursing as he or she progresses through the process of becoming a nurse leader. This was by no means intended to be an exhaustive discussion of every prominent nursing theorist but will hopefully pique the interest of the new registered nurse to do additional research. Many of the reviewed theorists have models they developed that use their specific concepts.

The process of developing into a nurse leader includes acquiring the knowledge needed to guide change when it must occur in an organization, and many of the theories addressed here could prove foundational to such a process. The details of the change process itself and how the registered nurse can successfully function as a change agent are discussed in the next chapter.

Critical Thinking Questions

1. Consider Virginia Henderson's theory of nursing.
   a. Discuss the major assumptions of this theory.
   b. Does this theory include a relationship to health? If so, describe the relationship.
   c. Does this theory include a relationship to the nursing process? If so, describe the relationship.
   d. Does this theory include a relationship to the environment? If so, describe the relationship.

2. Consider Imogene King's theory of nursing.
   a. Discuss the major assumptions of this theory.
   b. Does this theory include a relationship to health? If so, describe the relationship.
   c. Does this theory include a relationship to the nursing process? If so, describe the relationship.
   d. Does this theory include a relationship to the environment? If so, describe the relationship.

3. Consider Madeleine Leininger's theory of nursing.
   a. Discuss the major assumptions of this theory.
   b. Does this theory include a relationship to health? If so, describe the relationship.
   c. Does this theory include a relationship to the nursing process? If so, describe the relationship.
   d. Does this theory include a relationship to the environment? If so, describe the relationship.

4. Consider Betty Neuman's theory of nursing.
   a. Discuss the major assumptions of this theory.
   b. Does this theory include a relationship to health? If so, describe the relationship.
   c. Does this theory include a relationship to the nursing process? If so, describe the relationship.
   d. Does this theory include a relationship to the environment? If so, describe the relationship.

5. Consider Florence Nightingale's theory of nursing.
   a. Discuss the major assumptions of this theory.
   b. Does this theory include a relationship to health? If so, describe the relationship.
   c. Does this theory include a relationship to the nursing process? If so, describe the relationship.
   d. Does this theory include a relationship to the environment? If so, describe the relationship.
6. Consider Dorothea Orem's theory of nursing.
   a. Discuss the major assumptions of this theory.
   b. Does this theory include a relationship to health? If so, describe the relationship.
   c. Does this theory include a relationship to the nursing process? If so, describe the relationship.
   d. Does this theory include a relationship to the environment? If so, describe the relationship.
7. Consider Ida Orlando's theory of nursing.
   a. Discuss the major assumptions of this theory.
   b. Does this theory include a relationship to health? If so, describe the relationship.
   c. Does this theory include a relationship to the nursing process? If so, describe the relationship.
   d. Does this theory include a relationship to the environment? If so, describe the relationship.
8. Consider Hildegard Peplau's theory of nursing.
   a. Discuss the major assumptions of this theory.
   b. Does this theory include a relationship to health? If so, describe the relationship.
   c. Does this theory include a relationship to the nursing process? If so, describe the relationship.
   d. Does this theory include a relationship to the environment? If so, describe the relationship.
9. Consider Martha Rogers' theory of nursing.
   a. Discuss the major assumptions of this theory.
   b. Does this theory include a relationship to health? If so, describe the relationship.
   c. Does this theory include a relationship to the nursing process? If so, describe the relationship.

    d. Does this theory include a relationship to the environment? If so, describe the relationship.

10. Consider Sister Callista Roy's theory of nursing.

    a. Discuss the major assumptions of this theory.

    b. Does this theory include a relationship to health? If so, describe the relationship.

    c. Does this theory include a relationship to the nursing process? If so, describe the relationship.

    d. Does this theory include a relationship to the environment? If so, describe the relationship.

Scenarios

1. Discuss a situation in which you envision yourself using Virginia Henderson's theory of nursing in patient care.

    a. Has there ever been a time in your current job when you now realize Henderson's theory of nursing could have been used to explain a situation? If so, describe it in detail.

    b. If this theory could not have been used, is there a different theory of nursing that could have been useful at the time?

2. Discuss a situation when you can envision yourself using Imogene King's theory of nursing in patient care.

    a. Has there ever been a time in your current job when you now realize King's theory of nursing could have been used to explain a situation? If so, describe it in detail.

    b. If this theory could not have been used, is there a different theory of nursing that could have been useful at the time?

3. Discuss a situation in which you envision yourself using Madeleine Leininger's theory of nursing in patient care.

    a. Has there ever been a time in your current job when you now realize Leininger's theory of nursing could have been used to explain a situation? If so, describe it in detail.

    b. If this theory could not have been used, is there a different theory of nursing that could have been useful at the time?

4. Discuss a situation when you can envision yourself using Betty Neuman's theory of nursing in patient care.

    a. Has there ever been a time in your current job when you now realize Neuman's theory of nursing could have been used to explain a situation? If so, describe it in detail.

    b. If this theory could not have been used, is there a different theory of nursing that could have been useful at the time?

5. Discuss a situation in which you envision yourself using Florence Nightingale's theory of nursing in patient care.

    a. Has there ever been a time in your current job when you now realize Nightingale's theory of nursing could have been used to explain a situation? If so, describe it in detail.

    b. If this theory could not have been used, is there a different theory of nursing that could have been useful at the time?

6. Discuss a situation in which you envision yourself using Dorothea Orem's theory of nursing in patient care.

    a. Has there ever been a time in your current job when you now realize Orem's theory of nursing could have been used to explain a situation? If so, describe it in detail.

    b. If this theory could not have been used, is there a different theory of nursing that could have been useful at the time?

7. Discuss a situation when you can envision yourself using Ida Orlando's theory of nursing in patient care.

    a. Has there ever been a time in your current job when you now realize Orlando's theory of nursing could have been used to explain a situation? If so, describe it in detail.

    b. If this theory could not have been used, is there a different theory of nursing that could have been useful at the time?

8. Discuss a situation in which you envision yourself using Hildegard Peplau's theory of nursing in patient care.

    a. Has there ever been a time in your current job when you now realize Peplau's theory of nursing could have been used to explain a situation? If so, describe it in detail.

    b. If this theory could not have been used, is there a different theory of nursing that could have been useful at the time?

9. Discuss a situation when you can envision yourself using Martha Rogers' theory of nursing in patient care.

    a. Has there ever been a time in your current job when you now realize Rogers' theory of nursing could have been used to explain a situation? If so, describe it in detail.

    b. If this theory could not have been used, is there a different theory of nursing that could have been useful at the time?

10. Discuss a situation in which you can envision yourself using Sister Callista Roy's theory of nursing in patient care.

a. Has there ever been a time in your current job when you now realize Roy's theory of nursing could have been used to explain a situation? If so, describe it in detail.

b. If this theory could not have been used, is there a different theory of nursing that could have been useful at the time?

11. Select one of the nursing theories discussed in this chapter that appeals to you the most. Discuss why this particular theory appeals to you and how you will apply it in your daily nursing practice.

12. Compare and contrast Nightingale's theory of nursing with Orem's theory of nursing.

13. Compare and contrast King's theory of nursing with Neuman's theory of nursing.

14. Compare and contrast Rogers' theory of nursing with Roy's theory of nursing.

15. Compare and contrast Orlando's theory of nursing with Peplau's theory of nursing.

NCLEX® Questions

Using the information you obtained from studying this chapter, go online to complete the following NCLEX®-format review questions. Visit http://go.jblearning.com/terryLPN using the access code in the front cover of your book. This interactive resource allows you to answer each question and instantly review your results. Practice until you can answer at least 75% successfully, and then try to improve your score with each successive attempt.

Select the nursing theory that contains the following concepts.

1. _____ nursing, individual, health, environment

2. _____ ethnicity, acculturation, cultural awareness, cultural congruent care

3. _____ human being, intrapersonal stressors, interpersonal stressors, extrapersonal stressors

4. _____ distress, nursing role, nursing actions, outcome, nursing, outcome, nursing client

5. _____ stranger, teacher, resource person, counselor, surrogate, leader

6. _____ unitary human being, energy field, scope of nursing, health

7. _____ adaptation, focal stimuli, contextual stimuli, residual stimuli

a. Roy's theory

   b. Rogers' theory

   c. Leininger's theory

   d. Peplau's theory

   e. Henderson's theory

   f. Orem's theory

   g. Orlando's theory

   h. Neuman's theory

8. Documentation of the interaction that occurs between concepts and the patterns that result from that interaction form a

   a. proposition

   b. process

   c. model

   d. conceptual framework

9. Statements that explain relationships between the concepts used in a certain theory form a

   a. proposition

   b. process

   c. model

   d. conceptual framework

10. A series of actions, proposed changes, or functions that are implemented to bring about a specific result form a

   a. proposition

   b. process

   c. model

   d. conceptual framework

11. Functions that are basic needs of the individual according to Henderson's theory include

   a. financial stability

   b. cultural competence

   c. verbalizing thoughts

   d. participating in recreation

12. Madeleine Leininger's theory of nursing is based on the science of

   a. psychology

   b. sociology

   c. anthropology

   d. pathophysiology

13. According to Leininger's theory, the belief that members of a minority group usually assume the beliefs, practices, and values of the dominant cultural group in the society so that a blending of the cultural group occurs is known as
    a. ethnicity
    b. acculturation
    c. cultural awareness
    d. culturally congruent care

14. According to Leininger's theory, the awareness of belonging to a specific group is known as
    a. ethnicity
    b. acculturation
    c. cultural awareness
    d. culturally congruent care

15. According to Leininger's theory, _____ exists when the nurse examines his or her own background to assist in recognizing the existence of biases, prejudices, and assumptions that are present about other people.
    a. ethnicity
    b. acculturation
    c. cultural awareness
    d. culturally congruent care

16. Which one of the subtheories that compose Orem's theory of nursing explained why individuals can be helped through nursing?
    a. theory of self-care
    b. theory of self-care deficit
    c. theory of nursing systems
    d. theory of diagnostic operations

17. Which one of the subtheories that compose Orem's theory of nursing described why the individual will choose to care for him- or herself?
    a. theory of self-care
    b. theory of self-care deficit
    c. theory of nursing systems
    d. theory of diagnostic operations

18. Which one of the subtheories that compose Orem's theory of nursing proposed relationships that must be both developed and maintained in order for nursing to be implemented?
    a. theory of self-care

    b. theory of self-care deficit

    c. theory of nursing systems

    d. theory of diagnostic operations

19. Which one of the subtheories that compose Orem's theory of nursing described how care provided to the individual through nursing can be beneficial?

    a. theory of self-care

    b. theory of self-care deficit

    c. theory of nursing systems

    d. theory of diagnostic operations

20. Which one of the subtheories that compose Orem's theory of nursing attempted to explain the nature of the relationships that must be both developed and maintained in order for nursing to be implemented?

    a. theory of self-care

    b. theory of self-care deficit

    c. theory of nursing systems

    d. theory of diagnostic operations

For more information on the topics in this chapter and others, please see Appendix on p. 299 for a list of web linkss to additional resources.

References

Alligood, M., & Tomey, A. (2006). *Nursing theory: Utilization and application* (3rd ed.). Philadelphia, PA: Elsevier.

Chinn, P., & Kramer, M. (2010). *Integrated theory and knowledge development in nursing*. St. Louis, MO: Elsevier.

Chitty, K., & Black, B. (2007). *Professional nursing: Concepts and challenges* (5th ed.). Philadelphia, PA: Elsevier.

McElwen, M., & Wills, E. (2010). *Theoretical basis for nursing*. Philadelphia, PA: Lippincott, Williams, and Wilkins.

McKenna, H. (2002). *Nursing theories and models*. New York, NY: Routledge.

Parker, M., & Smith, M. (2010). *Nursing theories and nursing practice*. New York, NY: F. A. Davis.

Reed, P., & Shearer, N. (2011). *Perspectives on nursing theory*. Philadelphia, PA: Lippincott, Williams, and Wilkins.

Tomey, A., & Alligood, M. (2006). *Nursing theorists and their work* (6th ed.). Philadelphia, PA: Elsevier.

For a full suite of assignments and additional learning activities, use the access code located in the front of your book to visit this exclusive website: http://go. jblearning.com/terryLPN. If you do not have an access code, you can obtain one at the site.

CHAPTER OBJECTIVES

At the end of this chapter, you will be able to:

1. Discuss how the registered nurse can function as a change agent in the work setting.
2. Describe Lewin's theory of change.
3. Discuss what occurs in the process of change.
4. Discuss how the registered nurse can recognize and overcome resistance to change in the work setting.
5. Describe the registered nurse's personal response to the change process.

KEY TERMS

change agent
continuous change
decisive decision-making
developmental change
early adopter
early majority
emergent change
episodic change
evaluating
feedback
flexible decision-making
Force-Field Model of
    Change
hierarchic decision-making

implementing
informal change agent
innovator
integrative decision-
    making
intuitive decision-making
laggard
late majority
moving stage
negative feedback
organizing
participative or consensus
    decision-making
planned change

planning
refreezing stage
rejector
systematic decision-
    making
team decision-making
transformational change
transitional change
unfreezing stage
unilateral decision-making
vision

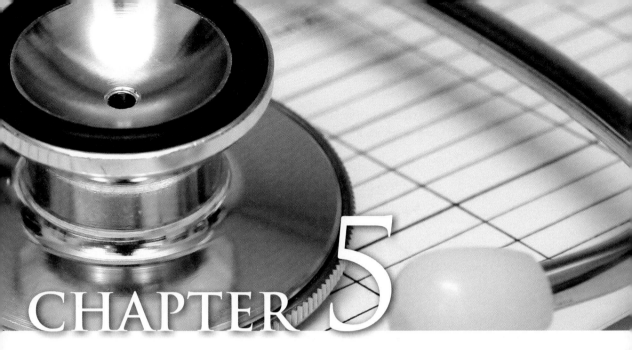

CHAPTER 5

Change Process

Introduction to the Change Process

Change is an inevitable part of the human experience, and as a nurse leader the registered nurse must have a clear understanding of how to recognize when change is needed in the work setting, the ways in which resistance can occur in response to change, how to successfully implement the change process, and, subsequently, how to recognize when change has been incorporated into the work setting and therefore can result in improved healthcare delivery. The nurse leader who has an integral understanding of the change process can function as a *change agent* to lead staff in implementing the process.

Change as a Concept

It is important for the nurse leader to thoroughly understand change because of its disruption of the equilibrium of the work environment. Such disruption tends to create tension in employees who already function in the high-stress arena of the modern healthcare facility. Therefore, the nurse leader must be able to recognize when employees are responding ineffectively to change and when he or she as a leader is not functioning appropriately as a change agent to facilitate the process. Staff can be frustrated by leadership that can neither cope effectively with the inevitable change that occurs in organizations nor facilitate the change as a seamless process. Change occurs so frequently in the modern healthcare facility due to a multitude of factors (Finkelman, 2012):

< New laws and regulations
< Modern technology
< Changes in the economy
< Healthcare reimbursement
< Changes in competition between facilities
< Changes in healthcare providers
< Medicare and Medicaid
< Nurse practice acts

Change Theory

Multiple theories have been developed regarding the process of change and how it unfolds in an organization, but one of the oldest and most used is Lewin's theory, which he referred to as the *Force-Field Model of Change*. Lewin's theory consists of three stages (Finkelman, 2012) (**Table 5-1**):

< *Unfreezing stage*: Focuses on developing awareness of the problem and recognizing and decreasing the forces that maintain the status quo. This includes determining if the problem can be improved by the proposed change. The unfreezing stage should produce a clear understanding of the issue at hand and can be the result of any type of employee meeting in which discussion is encouraged about the problem.

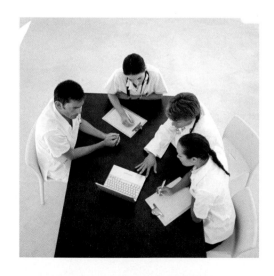

< *Moving stage*: Focuses on clearly identifying the issue at hand, developing goals and objectives, and developing and implementing strategies to meet the goals. This stage includes the development and encouragement of new values, attitudes, and behavior toward the proposed change.
< *Refreezing stage*: Occurs when the change has become part of the work environment. The goal for this stage is to prevent a return to past behavior patterns that resisted the change from occurring. It is not unusual in the modern healthcare delivery system for a facility to experience the refreezing stage of a change while simultaneously moving into another stage of a separate change process.

TABLE 5-1 **Phases of Lewin's Force-Field Model of Change**

Phase of Model	Description
Unfreezing	Focuses on developing awareness of the problem that is present and recognizing and decreasing the forces that are trying to maintain the status quo. This includes determining if the problem that is present can be improved by the proposed change. Should produce a clear understanding of the issue at hand; can be the result of an employee meeting in which discussion is encouraged about the problem.
Moving	Focuses on clearly identifying the issue at hand, the development of goals and objectives, and the development and implementation of strategies to meet the goals. This stage includes the development and encouragement of new values, attitudes, and behavior toward the proposed change.
Refreezing	Occurs when the change has become part of the work environment. The goal for this stage is to prevent a return to the past behavior patterns that resisted the change from occurring. A facility may experience the refreezing stage of a change while simultaneously moving into another stage of a separate change process.

Source: Finkelman, 2012.

Process of Change

Once the theory of how change unfolds is understood, the actual process of how it can be implemented in an organization can be reviewed. The nurse leader should implement the following process to successfully implement change in an organization (**Table 5-2**):

1. Motivate staff to make the change.
   - Staff must believe change is necessary but not so critical that it occurs too quickly. If the change progresses too quickly, the organization and staff may not be able to respond appropriately and the functioning of the organization may be jeopardized.
2. Seek staff support for the change.
   - Develop a group of staff to help build the momentum to implement the change.
3. Share the vision for the change with staff.
   - The *vision* is the basic concept that provides direction to implementation of the change. The staff should agree on the vision

TABLE 5-2 Stages of the Process of Change

Stage of the Change Process	Description of the Change Process
Motivate staff to make the change.	Staff must feel that change is necessary but not so critical that the change occurs too quickly. If the change progresses too quickly, the functioning of the organization may be jeopardized.
Seek staff support for the change.	Develop a group of staff to build the momentum to implement change.
Share the vision for the change with staff.	The vision is the concept that directs implementation of the change. The staff should agree on the vision for the future and then should be given the objectives that have been developed to reach the outcome. In order for staff to share the vision for the change, the nurse leader must be able to communicate clearly.
Empower staff to do what is necessary to make the change.	Staff members must be empowered in order to actively participate in making the change. The empowered staff member has been given the power to act. It is during this stage that any barriers such as resistance to change are identified and overcome in order to make the process occur more smoothly.
Develop short-term, measureable goals.	Although implementation of the change may be a lengthy process, the change agent should develop short-term, measureable goals so that staff can see that progress is being made and the change will be successful. The short-term, measurable goals serve as benchmarks for the change project.
Use this change as a springboard to produce additional change.	Once the change actually begins to take place and gains momentum, there is a tendency to allow the process to slow and to remove the focus from the need to accomplish the ultimate goal. Emphasize to staff the need to maintain small changes that are occurring along the way to accomplishing the most organizational-wide change. If the change process is allowed to stop too early before the final goal is accomplished, it will actually interfere with future change projects in the organization.

Stage of the Change Process	Description of the Change Process
Ensure that the values of the organization are reflective of the change that has occurred.	The change that is being implemented must be congruent with the values of the organization in order for the change to be implemented successfully. If the values are not congruent with the proposed change, the values must be very carefully changed.
Measure the success of the implemented change.	Use the measurable goals developed in the previous stages of the change to measure the overall success of the change once it is finalized. The change process must be monitored continuously so that adjustments can be made as necessary in the vision in preparation for future changes.

Source: Finkelman, 2012.

for the future and then should be given the objectives that have been developed to reach the outcome.

< For staff to share the vision for the change, the nurse leader must be able to communicate clearly. This includes informing all staff members of the aspects of the change, including expectations about how it will be implemented, and maintaining the approachability of the nurse leader.

< To implement the change accurately, staff must believe they can discuss the details of the change process as needed with the nurse leader. In turn, the nurse leader must demonstrate active listening and patience to indicate he or she hears staff members' concerns even when they may initially contradict the leader's vision (Morjikian, Kimball, & Joynt, 2007).

4. Empower staff to do what is necessary to make the change.

< Staff members must be empowered to actively participate in making the change. It is during this stage that any barriers such as resistance to change are identified and overcome to make the process occur more smoothly.

5. Develop short-term, measurable goals.

< Although implementation of the change is a process that may prove to be lengthy, the change agent should develop short-term, measurable

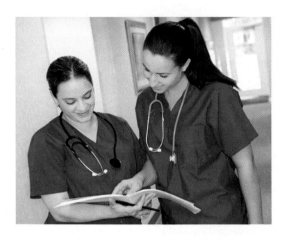

goals so the staff can see that progress is being made and incorporation of the change will be successful.

< The short-term, measurable goals are particularly important because they serve as benchmarks for the change project, allowing the change agent to determine at any point in the process if everything is progressing as originally intended.

6. Use this change as a springboard to produce additional change.

< Once the change actually begins to take place and gains momentum, there is a tendency to allow the process to slow and to remove the focus from the need to accomplish the ultimate goal.

< Emphasize to staff the need to maintain the small changes that occur along the way to accomplishing the most significant organizational-wide change.

< If the change process is allowed to stop too early before the final goal is accomplished, it will actually interfere with future change projects in the organization. Staff may gain the impression the facility does not implement changes completely and smoothly and may try to avoid participating in future change projects.

7. Ensure the values of the organization are reflective of the change that has occurred.

< The proposed change must be congruent with the values of the organization for the change to be implemented successfully.

< If the values are not congruent with the proposed change, the values must be very carefully changed. For example, if the facility proposes a change from primary to team nursing in an effort to increase staff efficiency and effectiveness and is soliciting staff input on the decision, a value shift will need to occur if the facility has not shown a willingness to incorporate staff suggestions before this point.

8. Measure the success of the implemented change.

< Use the measurable goals developed in the previous stages of the change to measure the overall success of the change once it is finalized. The change process must be monitored continuously so adjustments can be made as necessary in the vision in preparation for future changes (Finkelman, 2012).

Registered Nurse as a Change Agent

The registered nurse who is as a change agent uses his or her knowledge base and skill set to either lead the change process or to influence the change and to simultaneously contribute to trust development in the staff members involved in the process. Because the change agent will be working with both human and technological elements in the change process, which both may prove to be unpredictable at times, the agent must be well versed in the ability to interact successfully with others, maintain flexibility in crisis situations, choose the most appropriate timing of crucial decisions, and manage conflict at the most basic level of the change process.

Some change processes may be complicated enough to benefit from the assistance of an *informal change agent* who will work closely with the formal change agent. The informal change agent can bring his or her expertise and positive attitude toward the proposed change to the process for staff members who are still uncertain about the change, thus reinforcing the great benefit for both the organization and staff.

Finally, the informal change agent can be invaluable to the formal change agent in identifying and overcoming resistance to the proposed change. Morjikian and colleagues (2007) noted the less resistance to a proposed change in an organization, the more likely it is a fairly insignificant change with minimal impact on the facility itself. Therefore, resistance to the change process should be both expected and identified early enough to be rendered ineffective (Yoder-Wise, 2007).

Change Management Functions of the Change Agent

The change agent has five primary management functions to assist in the implementation of change to achieve a specific goal (Yoder-Wise, 2007). The functions may be used in any sequence and may in fact be used simultaneously if the particular change process would be strengthened by the use of multiple functions. The five functions are as follows:

< Planning
< Organizing
< Implementing

‹ Evaluating

‹ Seeking feedback

Planning consists of looking ahead to decide on the most effective way to achieve a preset goal. For the plan to be effective, both the change agent implementing the plan and the people affected by the change must take part in the process of planning for the change to occur. Factors that will most likely favor or resist the progress of the change must be thoroughly assessed. It may help to clarify plans for a change process by documenting general information gained in the planning process so participants can understand their future roles and responsibilities (Yoder-Wise, 2007). Morjikian et al. (2007) noted that the formal planning process should include at the very least the development of important assumptions, strategies, operating requirements, resource needs, financial analysis, and contingency strategies.

Organizing involves decision-making using resources in the form of time, personnel, communication, or raw materials. This function of the change agent involves weighing the pros and cons of various options to achieve maximum efficiency. Organizing is an important function because it solidifies the resources to be used in generating the change (Yoder-Wise, 2007). The change agent who is able to organize appropriately will recognize the most effective strategy in producing the highest quality work performance from each employee. Organizing includes acquiring an intimate understanding of the inner workings of the organization, recognizing how to use both formal and informal channels to accomplish the goals set as part of the change process, understanding the rationale behind the organization's policies and procedures, and recognizing the key points in the organizational culture (Morjikian et al., 2007).

Implementing usually occurs after the plan is established. However, an unexpected change may require immediate implementation and subsequently a rapid change in the plan. The nature of change is such that an alteration in one part of a system can affect the management function in other systems that may 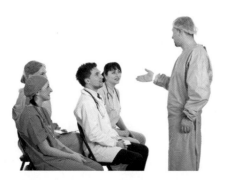 be related (Yoder-Wise, 2007). Morjikian and coworkers (2007) noted that implementation of the change process may proceed more smoothly if the nurse leader has a strong personal presence. The leader with a charismatic personality is more likely to make the informal connections with other leaders needed to make a change in a multilayered organization.

Evaluating is a vital part of the management functions because it involves a judgment of the extent to which the change process is progressing toward the intended outcome.

The change agent should continuously monitor the change process to detect any problems that occur and to make any needed adjustments to avoid a failure of the process (Yoder-Wise, 2007). If the change agent detects a problem, a rapid adjustment will need to be made, and thus the implementation function may simultaneously function to resolve the issue.

The change agent seeks out *feedback* on the change that is being implemented by a continuous process of data gathering. Some of the most important information is gained through review of *negative feedback*. Negative feedback is information that indicates the existence of a problem and the need to make a correction to either continue the progress being made in the change process or to refocus the process so that it is congruent with the original intended outcome (Yoder-Wise, 2007).

The nurse leader in the position of change agent should have a knowledge base of the management functions and skill set to strengthen the process of a proposed change. A change agent who determines a change process has either slowed or deviated from its desired outcome should consider if all the management functions have been used appropriately (**Table 5-3**).

TABLE 5-3 Change Management Functions of the Change Agent

Function	Description	Actions of the Change Agent
Planning	Consists of looking ahead to decide on the most effective way to achieve a preset goal.	In order for the plan to be effective, both change agent and the people affected by the change must take part in the planning process. Factors that will favor or resist the progress of the change must be assessed.
Organizing	Involves making decisions using resources such as time, personnel, communication, or raw materials. This function of the change agent involves weighing the pros and cons of various options in order to achieve maximum efficiency.	The change agent who is able to organize appropriately will be able to recognize which strategy will produce the highest quality work performance from each employee. Organizing includes understanding the inner workings of the organization, recognizing how to use formal and informal channels to accomplish goals, understanding the rationale behind policies and procedures, and recognizing key points in the organizational culture.

Function	Description	Actions of the Change Agent
Implementing	Usually occurs after the plan is established, although an unexpected change may require immediate implementation and a rapid change in the plan.	Implementation of the change process may proceed more smoothly if the nurse leader has a strong personal presence; a charismatic leader is more likely to be able to make the informal connections that will be needed to make a change in a multi-layered organization.
Evaluating	Involves judging extent to which change process is progressing toward the intended outcome.	The change agent should continuously monitor the change process to detect problems that are occurring and make any needed adjustments to avoid failure of the process.
Feedback	Involves a continuous data gathering process.	The change agent can gain some of the most important information through review of negative feedback.

Source: Yoder-Wise, 2007; Morjikian, Kimball, & Joynt, 2007.

Responding to Change

A change agent needs to understand the human response to the change process. Initial responses to change are most typically reluctance and resistance. These responses are usually due to the threat to personal security generated by the change process. In addition, the change process generally produces one of six behavioral responses (Yoder-Wise, 2007):

< The *innovator* enjoys change but may not completely comprehend the degree of instability that can be created in the workplace environment by change; this person will be completely supportive of the change agent's actions but may try to move the process too quickly in his or her enthusiasm.
< The *early adopter* is consulted regarding information about changes because of the high esteem with which they are held by their colleagues. This person can be one of the greatest allies of the change agent.
< The *early majority* has a preference for what was done in the past but will accept the new status quo created by the change. This person will be supportive of the actions of the change agent but may be reluctant to move the change process too quickly or to make more than incremental changes.

< The *late majority* is open about his or her negative feelings about the change and agrees to accept it only after others have accepted and incorporated it. This person will demonstrate resistance to the actions of the change agent and may be passive-aggressive in response.

< The *laggard* would rather continue to practice traditional methods and openly acknowledges his or her resistance to new ideas. This person will demonstrate resistance to the actions of the change agent and may be passive-aggressive in response.

< The *rejector* chooses to actively oppose change and may even sabotage the progress toward a positive outcome. This person will be a challenge to the change agent because of his or her open resistance. The change agent may require the collaboration of other nurse leaders if this individual becomes particularly aggressive.

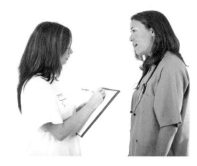

The change agent must understand not only the behavioral responses to change but also their underlying motives because this will be the key to winning employees' support for the proposed change (**Table 5-4**). Perhaps most

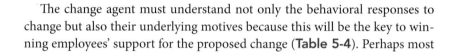

TABLE 5-4 Behavioral Responses to the Change Process

Behavioral Response	Description	Relationship to the Change Agent
Innovator	Enjoys change but may not completely comprehend degree of instability created in the workplace environment by change.	Completely supportive of the change agent's actions but may try to move the process too quickly in his or her enthusiasm.
Early adopter	Consulted about change occurring because of high esteem with which they are held by peers.	Can be important ally of the change agent.
Early majority	Prefers what was done in the past but will accept new status quo created by the change.	Support actions of change agent but may hesitate to move process too quickly or make more than incremental changes.
Late majority	Negative feelings about change; will accept after others have accepted and incorporated it.	Shows resistance to the actions of the change agent and may be passive-aggressive in response.

Behavioral Response	Description	Relationship to the Change Agent
Laggard	Would prefer practice traditional methods; acknowledges resistance to new ideas.	Shows resistance to the actions of the change agent and may be passive-aggressive in response.
Rejector	Actively oppose change; may sabotage progress made toward a positive outcome.	Will be a challenge due to open resistance; assistance of other nurse leaders may be needed.

Source: Yoder-Wise, 2007.

importantly of all, the change agent must understand his or her own behavioral response to change to ensure the response is congruent with the desire outcome of the change process and not inadvertently hostile to it.

Forms of Change

In addition to both the theoretical basis for change and the basic process of change, management functions to expedite change. In the role of change agent, the registered nurse must have an understanding of the behavioral responses that can occur as a result of change and of the type of change that is occurring (**Table 5-5**). According to Redfern and Christian (2003), several types of change can be used in an organization:

- *Planned change*: This involves logical action that is based on deliberate reasoning and usually includes a formal change agent who is well versed in the change process.
- *Emergent change*: This change occurs spontaneously; it is unplanned and subsequently may be unable to be controlled and may not involve a change agent.
- *Episodic change*: This change occurs because it was planned and is intended to occur on an occasional basis.
- *Continuous change*: This type of change occurs on an incremental basis so that it is always evolving toward the final intended outcome. The results of each incremental change are cumulative.
- *Developmental change*: This change can be either planned or emergent and, like continuous change, develops incrementally over time.

TABLE 5-5 Forms of Change

Form of Change	Description	Change Agent Used
Planned change	Involves logical action that is based on deliberate reasoning	Usually implemented with a change agent
Emergent change	Change that occurs spontaneously; it is unplanned and subsequently may be unable to be controlled	May not involve a change agent because of the spontaneous nature of the change
Episodic change	Occurs because it was planned and is intended to occur on an occasional basis	Will usually involve a change agent
Continuous change	Occurs on an incremental basis so that it is always evolving toward the final intended outcome; the results of each incremental change are cumulative	More likely to involve an informal rather than formal change agent because of the constant evolving nature of the change
Developmental change	Can be either planned or emergent, and like continuous change, develops incrementally over time;	May involve a change agent if it is planned
Transitional change	Occurs in planned episodes and usually is radical in nature;	May be difficult to implement without a change agent because of the radical nature of the change
Transformational change	Like transitional change, considered to be radical in nature; like emergent change, may be uncontrolled during the period of time that it takes the change to develop; the new changed condition will develop after the deterioration of the old condition	May not involve a change agent because of the radical and uncontrolled nature of the change

Source: Redfern & Christian, 2003.

< *Transitional change*: This occurs in planned episodes and usually is radical in nature.

< *Transformational change*: Like transitional change, this is considered to be radical in nature and, like emergent change, may be uncontrolled during the time it takes the change to develop. The new changed condition will develop after the deterioration of the old condition.

If the change agent can specify the type of change, he or she can assist with the change process and particularly evaluate the progress being made toward the ultimate intended outcome.

Responding to Change

In most cases the result of the change process is decision-making. Just as there is a process to the formation of change, there is also a process to decision-making. In this case it begins with a problem being identified and ends with the weighing of the merits of various choices and a course of action being selected. Decision-making is an integral part of the planning phase of the change process and a direct response to change. Various styles of decision-making can be used by a change agent and collaborating nurse leaders throughout the change process and at the conclusion of the process (Finkelman, 2012) (**Table 5-6**):

- < *Unilateral*: This consists of one person making a decision with limited input from other colleagues. This style usually does not work well in a

TABLE 5-6 **Styles of Decision-Making**

Style of Decision-Making	Description	Effective with a Change Agent
Unilateral	This style consists of one person making a decision with limited input from other colleagues.	This style usually does not work well in a large healthcare organization with multiple stakeholders who are all affected by any type of decision as well as the smallest incremental change.
Participative or Consensus	This style consists of actively attempting to involve others in the decision-making process, even if the decision is such that one individual must make the final decision.	This style works well with a change agent monitoring the change process.
Decisive	This style does not require a large amount of available information in order to make a decision.	This style can be utilized with a change agent.

Style of Decision-Making	Description	Effective with a Change Agent
Integrative	This style uses all available data in the decision-making process and identifies multiple alternatives that can be utilized in arriving at a final decision.	This style can be used successfully with a change agent.
Hierarchic	This style will utilize a large amount of information in making the decision but will identify one solution or one alternative to be generated.	This style can be used successfully with a change agent.
Flexible	This style will utilize a small amount of data in decision-making, produces multiple alternatives, and may result in a change in the final decision if additional information is revealed or available information is reinterpreted.	This style can be used successfully with a change agent.
Systematic	This style utilizes a structured approach to making decisions and a logical approach to forming the final decision.	This style can be used successfully with a change agent.
Intuitive	This style uses a trial-and-error approach to decision-making.	This style does not work well with a change agent because it relies on focusing on the general feeling that the person derives from the alternative presented and tends to ignore available information.
Team	This style focuses on bringing together collaborators' multiple ideas and experiences to produce a result that is much more extensive than the individual pieces of information that generated the decision. This can be a very effective style of decision-making when there is need for additional ideas or alternatives.	This style can be used successfully with a change agent.

Source: Finkelman, 2012.

large healthcare organization with multiple stakeholders who are both affected by any type of decision as well as the smallest incremental change.

< *Participative* or *consensus*: This consists of actively attempting to involve others in the decision-making process, even if the decision is such that one individual must make the final decision. This style works well with one change agent who monitors the change process.

< *Decisive*: This does not require a large amount of available information to make a decision.

< *Integrative*: This uses all available data in the decision-making process and identifies multiple alternatives to arrive at a final decision.

< *Hierarchic*: This uses a large amount of information in making the decision but identifies one solution or one alternative.

< *Flexible*: This uses a small amount of data in decision-making, produces multiple alternatives, and may result in a change in the final decision if additional information is revealed or available information is reinterpreted.

< *Systematic*: A structured approach is used to making decisions and a logical approach to forming the final decision.

< *Intuitive*: This trial-and-error approach does not work well with a change agent because it relies on a focus on the general feeling one derives from the alternatives presented and tends to ignore available information.

< *Team*: This approach focuses on bringing together collaborators' multiple ideas and experiences to produce a result that is much more extensive than the individual pieces of information that generated the decision. This can be a very effective style of decision-making when there is need for additional ideas or alternatives to be generated.

Once the most effective decision-making style has been established, the types of decisions the change agent may be called on to make must be determined. Two major types of decisions are programmed decisions and nonprogrammed decisions. Programmed decisions typically are more routine, can be made relatively quickly, and usually are related to a policy or procedure of the facility. Nonprogrammed decisions are not typical and may in fact be crises. They usually require a large investment in data collection, analysis of the situation at hand, and collaboration with other nurse leaders and department heads. The nonprogrammed decision usually requires a considerable amount of nursing judgment because there may not be a precedent for making such a decision. Clearly, the skill set and knowledge base of the change agent can be used most effectively with the nonprogrammed decision (Finkelman, 2012).

Summary of Key Points in the Chapter

The nurse leader who functions as a change agent can be effective in guiding the decision-making process in an organization. The following are the major steps in the decision-making:

< Recognize the existence of a problem and define it in clear terms.
< Gather all relevant information that is available on the problem.
< Identify all possible solutions that could be used to resolve the problem.
< Assess the various solutions for their viability as a final resolution for the problem.
< Evaluate results of the assessment of the solution.
< Reach a decision regarding an ultimate solution to the problem.

The change agent can prove to be invaluable in guiding the organization through the decision-making process, particularly when a nonprogrammed decision is at stake (Finkelman, 2012).

This chapter discussed various aspects of the process of change:

< Process of change
< Forms of change that can occur
< Lewin's theory of change and the Force-Field Model
< Registered nurse change agent
< Management functions used by the change agent
< Decision-making as a response to change
< Styles of decision-making and the process of decision-making

Conclusion

The registered nurse leader in the position of change agent in an organization must have a clear understanding of how the process of change progresses as well as the management functions needed to expedite that process. The change agent who has that understanding will be prepared to respond appropriately to change by subsequently using the decision-making process.

Occasionally, changes involve a policy or procedure that is focused on health promotion and the specific levels of primary, secondary, and tertiary prevention. The next chapter discusses the concept of health promotion and how it affects the nurse leader in an organization.

Critical Thinking Questions

1. Many factors have been described as affecting change in the modern healthcare facility. Think about your own work setting. What factors do you recognize as having affected a change that occurred in your own work environment? Discuss why you believe each factor had an effect on the change in the work setting and what the effect was.

2. Consider the stages of Lewin's Force-Field Model of Change. Think of a time in your current or past work environment when you recognize the unfreezing stage of Lewin's Model occurred. Describe how the unfreezing stage occurred and the result of the stage.

3. Consider the stages of Lewin's Force-Field Model of Change. Think of a time in your current or past work environment when you recognize the moving stage of Lewin's Model occurred. Describe how the moving stage occurred and the result of the stage.

4. Consider the stages of Lewin's Force-Field Model of Change. Think of a time in your current or past work environment when you recognize the refreezing stage of Lewin's Model occurred. Describe how the refreezing stage occurred and the result of the stage.

5. Think about a change that was recently implemented in your current work setting. Can you identify the formal change agent? Describe how the change agent used planning and organizing as management functions to assist the change process. Was the change ultimately successful? If so, what actions on the part of the change agent helped promote the change? If not, did actions on the part of the change agent inadvertently hinder the change?

6. Think about a change that was recently implemented in your current work setting. Can you identify the formal change agent? Describe how the change agent used implementing and evaluating as management functions to assist the change process. Do you believe that these management functions were used successfully? Be able to support your answer.

7. Think about a change that was recently implemented in your current work setting. Can you identify the formal change agent? Describe how the change agent used feedback, particularly the gathering of negative feedback, as a management function to assist the change process. Do you believe this management function was used successfully? Be able to support your answer.

8. Analyze your own typical response to change. Which one of the six usual behavioral responses usually typifies you? Be able to support your answer.

9. Analyze your own decision-making style. What one of the nine decision-making styles most typifies you? Do you believe your current decision-making style will be helpful when you function as a change agent? Be able to support your answer.

10. You are functioning as the change agent for an organization. At the conclusion of a change process a nonprogrammed decision must be made. Which style(s) of decision-making do you believe would assist the change agent most effectively in making a nonprogrammed decision? Be able to support your answer.

Scenarios

1. You are the unit manager of a 30-bed oncology floor. You receive a memo from hospital administration that the facility will be moving from 8-hour shifts to 12-hour shifts. Consider Lewin's Force-Field Model of Change. Use each stage of the model to describe how it could be used to implement this particular change.

2. You are the unit manager of a 30-bed oncology floor. You receive a memo from hospital administration that the facility will be moving from 8-hour shifts to 12-hour shifts. Consider the stages in the process of change. How can you motivate staff to make the change? How can you develop a group of staff to help build the momentum to implement the change?

3. You are the unit manager of a 30-bed oncology floor. You receive a memo from hospital administration that the facility will be moving from 8-hour shifts to 12-hour shifts. Consider the stages in the process of change. Describe the vision for the change as you would communicate it to staff members.

4. You are the unit manager of a 30-bed oncology floor. You receive a memo from hospital administration that the facility will be moving from 8-hour shifts to 12-hour shifts. Consider the stages in the process of change. How can you empower employees to assist in making the change? What type of resistance do you believe will be offered to try to prevent the change?

5. You are the unit manager of a 30-bed oncology floor. You receive a memo from hospital administration that the facility will be moving from 8-hour shifts to 12-hour shifts. Consider the stages in the process of change. Develop short-term, measurable goals for the change and describe how their accomplishment could be evaluated.

6. You are the unit manager of a 30-bed oncology floor. You receive a memo from hospital administration that the facility will be moving

from 8-hour shifts to 12-hour shifts. Consider the stages in the process of change. You find that progress is being made in implementing the change. What needs to be done to maintain the change that has occurred and to prevent the change that is still in progress from slowing?

7. You are the unit manager of a 30-bed oncology floor. You receive a memo from hospital administration that the facility will be moving from 8-hour shifts to 12-hour shifts. Consider the stages in the process of change. As the change is being implemented, staff are concerned the change will not be permanent because the nurses have asked for such a schedule change before and it was never implemented previously. How can you convince staff of the change in the values of the organization?

8. You are the unit manager of a 30-bed oncology floor. You receive a memo from hospital administration that the facility will be moving from 8-hour shifts to 12-hour shifts. Consider the stages in the process of change. How can you monitor the progress of the change once it has occurred? How can you determine if the vision for the change needs to be adjusted?

9. You are a staff nurse working on a 35-bed neuroscience floor. The unit manager tells you the facility is going to offer 12-hour weekend shifts as a staffing option. Describe how you could assist in the implementation of this change by functioning as an informal change agent.

10. Your hospital administration has made the decision to combine your 20-bed medical-surgical unit with a 15-bed cardiac step-down floor. The change is scheduled to be implemented over the next 3 months. What form of change do you believe this is? Based on the form of the change, do you believe a formal change agent should be involved? Describe the role of a formal change agent in this form of change.

11. The situation described in scenario 10 now must be implemented over the next 2 weeks because the hospital is scheduled to be sold to another healthcare company. Based on this new information, what form of change do you believe this is? Based on the form of the change, do you believe a formal change agent should be involved? Describe the role of a formal change agent in this form of change.

12. You are the unit manager in a large metropolitan hospital and will be serving as the formal change agent during a large-scale change process. You have determined that you have a hierarchic style of decision-making. You would like to use your assistant unit manager as an informal change agent during the process. However, the assistant unit manager has an intuitive decision-making style. Analyze this situation

and determine how you can most effectively work with the informal change agent during the change process.

13. You are the nurse administrator for a large metropolitan medical center. The hospital is scheduled to be remodeled. You must decide whether a 22-bed cardiac step-down floor should be closed for 6 weeks during the remodeling and place those employees in various areas throughout the hospital or have the floor combined with an adjacent 15-bed dialysis unit. If the floor and the dialysis unit combine, the cardiac floor's assistant nurse manager will supervise the combined area because both the floor and the unit are lacking a unit manager right now. This is a nonprogrammed decision and there is no precedent for something similar having ever happened in the facility. Which style of decision-making do you believe would be most effective? Be prepared to support your answer.

14. Review scenario 13. Work through the decision process step by step to show how you produced the decision that you made.

NCLEX® Review Questions

Using the information you obtained from studying this chapter, go online to complete the following NCLEX®-format review questions. Visit http://go.jblearning.com/terryLPN using the access code in the front cover of your book. This interactive resource allows you to answer each question and instantly review your results. Practice until you can answer at least 75% successfully, and then try to improve your score with each successive attempt.

Select the form of change that matches the description given.

1. _____ occurs in planned episodes; radical in nature
2. _____ can be planned or emergent; develops incrementally
3. _____ radical in nature; may be uncontrolled while change is developing
4. _____ occurs incrementally and is always evolving toward final intended outcome
5. _____ was planned and intended to occur on occasional basis
6. _____ logical action based on deliberate reasoning
7. _____ occurs spontaneously; may be unplanned and therefore unable to be controlled
   a. transformational change
   b. transitional change
   c. developmental change

d. continuous change

e. episodic change

f. emergent change

g. planned change

Select the change management function that matches the description.

8. _____ judging extent to which change process progresses toward intended outcome

9. _____ involves a continuous data-gathering process

10. _____ involves making decisions using resources

11. _____ occurs after plan is established; proceeds more smoothly with a strong leader

12. _____ involves weighing pros and cons of options to achieve maximum efficiency

13. _____ looking ahead to decide on most effective way to achieve preset goal

a. planning

b. organizing

c. implementing

d. evaluating

e. feedback

Select the response to change that corresponds to the description.

14. _____ preference for what was done in the past but will accept new status quo

15. _____ would rather continue to practice traditional methods; acknowledges resistance

16. _____ chooses to actively oppose change and may sabotage progress being made

17. _____ resists actions of change agent; may be passive-aggressive; openly negative

18. _____ can be one of the greatest allies of the change agent

19. _____ consulted about changes due to high esteem with which they are held colleagues

20. _____ may try to move the process too quickly because of his enthusiasm

a. laggard

b. rejector

c. late majority

d. early majority

e. early adopter

f. innovator

For more information on the topics in this chapter and others, please see Appendix on p. 299 for a list of web links to additional resources.

References

Finkelman, A. (2012). *Leadership and management for nurses* (2nd ed.). Boston, MA: Pearson.

Morjikian, R., Kimball, B., & Joynt, J. (2007). The nurse executive's role in implementing new care delivery models. *Journal of Nursing Administration, 37,* 399–404.

Redfern, S., & Christian, S. (2003). Achieving change in health care practice. *Journal of Evaluation in Clinical Practice, 9,* 225–238.

Yoder-Wise, P. (2007). *Leading and managing in nursing* (4th ed.). Philadelphia, PA: Elsevier.

For a full suite of assignments and additional learning activities, use the access code located in the front of your book to visit this exclusive website: http://go.jblearning.com/terryLPN. If you do not have an access code, you can obtain one at the site.

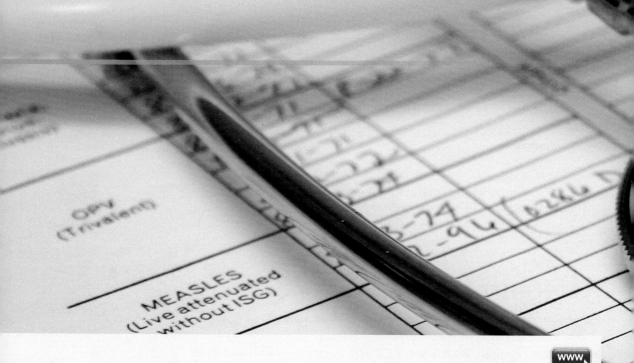

www

CHAPTER OBJECTIVES

At the end of this chapter, you will be able to:

1. Discuss screening and counseling as aspects of health promotion.
2. Describe the major aspects of the health belief model.
3. Describe the major aspects of Pender's health promotion model.
4. Compare and contrast primary, secondary, and tertiary prevention.
5. Describe the major aspects of the transtheoretical model of change.

www

KEY TERMS

action
challenge
commitment
contemplation
control
cues to action
general adaptation
    syndrome
hardiness
health belief model

health promotion
health risk appraisal
Healthy People 2020
maintenance
Pender's model of health
    promotion
perceived barriers
perceived benefit
perceived susceptibility
perceived threat

precontemplation
preparation
primary prevention
secondary prevention
self-efficacy
tertiary prevention
theoretical proposition
transtheoretical model of
    change

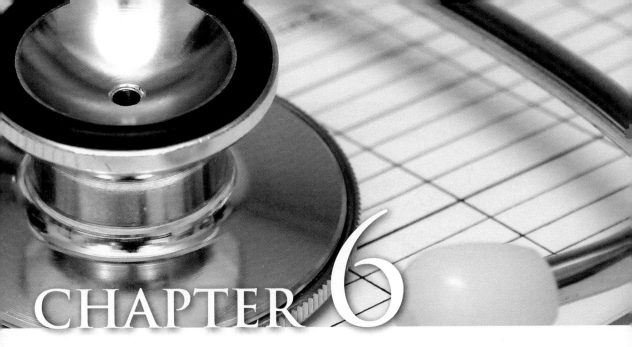

CHAPTER 6

Health Promotion

Introduction to Health Promotion

The nurse who is moving into the registered nurse role and who also aspires to become a nurse leader will need to become well-versed in how health care is financed in the modern era. Both insurers and Medicare are providing additional funding for health promotion strategies. *Health promotion* is important because it uses education to provide people with the knowledge needed to maintain their own health (**Table 6-1**). As healthcare insurers develop services for health promotion and disease prevention for patients, companies then reevaluate the costs and benefits of the services to people who are insured. Three primary types of health promotion and disease prevention methods currently used by healthcare insurers and organizations are as follows (Finkelman, 2012):

‹ Screening: A battery of laboratory tests, including annual physical examinations and laboratory testing, are selected based on a risk assessment of the patient. The risk assessment consists of an evaluation of the patient's medical history, family history, lifestyle practices such as smoking and alcohol usage, health maintenance practices such as regular exercise, and nutritional habits.

‹ Counseling: The healthcare professional explains the relationship between the patient's identified risk factors as determined by the risk

TABLE 6-1 Types of Health Promotion Activities

Health Promotion Activity	Description
Screening	This includes annual physical examinations and laboratory testing. The battery of laboratory tests selected will be based on a risk assessment of the patient. The risk assessment consists of an evaluation of the patient's medical history, family history, lifestyle practices, health maintenance practices, and nutritional habits.
Counseling	The nurse explains the relationship between patient's identified risk factors as determined by risk assessment and patient's overall health. Counseling is the tool by which the RN can help the patient develop the knowledge base, skill set and motivation to maintain their current level of health based on both acute and chronic disease processes and to acquire new health practices that will increase his level of health.
Immunization	The registered nurse will provide patients with the information needed to make decisions about their health and the health of their children.

Source: Finkelman, 2012.

assessment and the patient's overall level of health. Counseling is the tool by which the registered nurse can help the patient develop the knowledge base and skill set as well as the motivation to maintain his or her current level of health based on both acute and chronic disease processes and to acquire new health practices to increase the level of health.

< Immunization: The registered nurse provides patients with the information needed to make decisions about their health and the health of their children.

Health promotion is of such importance that the U.S. Department of Health and Human Services (2010) developed ***Healthy People 2020***. This initiative contains goals and objectives for America's health promotion and disease prevention and has provided a critical design for public health priorities and interventions for the past 30 years. Funds are allocated to develop programs that are aimed at identifying risk factors and preventing the development of chronic conditions such as cardiac disease, various forms of cancer, and diabetes mellitus. These chronic conditions cause 7 of 10 American deaths annually and result in 75% of American funds allocated toward health (U.S. Department of Health and Human Services, 2010).

Disease Prevention

Disease prevention is an aspect of health promotion. Three types of disease prevention strategies can be used (**Table 6-2**):

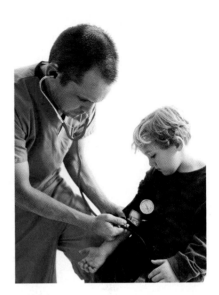

< *Primary prevention*: These interventions focus on behaviors that maintain wellness and prevent the development of illness and can include exercise classes, water safety classes, seminars on women's health, and heart-healthy meal planning.
< *Secondary prevention*: These interventions focus on diagnosing disease processes early, recognizing the existence of symptoms, and initiating treatment as rapidly as possible to avoid the development of complications.
< *Tertiary prevention*: These interventions focus on rehabilitation after the development of a disease to prevent disabling complications (Finkelman, 2012).

TABLE 6-2 Disease Prevention Strategies

Disease Prevention Strategy	Description	Example of Activity
Primary prevention	Focuses on behaviors that maintain wellness and prevent the development of illness	Interventions can include exercise classes, water safety classes, seminars on women's health, and heart-healthy meal planning
Secondary prevention	Focuses on diagnosing disease processes early, recognizing the existence of symptoms, and initiating treatment as rapidly as possible to avoid the development of complications	Interventions can include laboratory testing and x-rays performed as part of an attempt to diagnose the cause of symptoms
Tertiary prevention	Focuses on rehabilitation after the development of a disease with the intent of preventing disability	Interventions can include physically-based strategies such as physical therapy as well as emotionally-based strategies such as psychiatric therapy if the patient experienced trauma

Source: Finkelman, 2012.

According to Williams (2008), primary prevention is significant because of its low-cost approach to decreasing the likelihood of a healthy individual becoming an unhealthy one. Because a key component of this type of disease prevention is patient education, the registered nurse must assess patients thoroughly to provide them with accurate health maintenance information in their own language that is congruent with their current reading and comprehension levels. Primary prevention must include providing patients, particularly those from vulnerable populations, with information about the types of resources available to them in their home communities. Primary prevention programs that are implemented correctly can result in a decreased rate of mortality, decreased incidence of substance abuse, increased overall level of health in vulnerable populations such as children and the elderly, and an overall increased level of health, fitness, and well-being for entire communities (Williams, 2008).

Secondary prevention focuses on diagnosing disease processes early, recognizing the existence of symptoms as they develop, and initiating treatment as rapidly as possible to avoid the development of complications. This intent was implemented by Irmak and Fesci (2010), who designed a program for cardiac patients. The researchers initiated secondary prevention strategies in a hospital setting and continued them after discharge using home health care. Irmak and Fesci (2010) concluded that the secondary prevention strategies resulted in a decrease of the overall systolic and diastolic blood pressure, cholesterol level, and body mass index. In addition, the strategies directly resulted in a decrease in the number of patients who chose to continue smoking and an increase in the number of those who became more concerned about their eating habits as well as regular exercise.

Tertiary prevention, focusing on rehabilitation after significant illness, has been used with success with cancer survivors. In this population of patients it includes strategies to expedite the early detection of additional malignancies and to reduce the existence of risk factors for the development of secondary malignancies and long-term complications resulting from treatment options. Tertiary prevention measures are implemented when prognosis for cure is favorable and screening measures may result in an improved quality of life for the patient. Rehabilitation after a serious illness such as cancer should include educating the patient about the signs and symptoms of additional malignancies, the importance of a healthy lifestyle, and the need to be screened for various forms of cancer on a regular basis. Cancer survivors who have been educated in such a manner have been shown to be better advocates for themselves, more fully engaged in living with a diagnosis of cancer long term, and less stressed by the prospect of incorporating such a diagnosis into their daily life (Mahon, 2005).

Pender's Model of Health Promotion

Just as nursing theorists developed ideas to explain the origins of nursing as a profession, so have theorists proposed various models of health promotion. One of the best known was developed by Dr. Nola Pender and is unique for its view of health. *Pender's model of health promotion* proposes that health is a dynamic state, ever in transition, and thus health promotion should strive to constantly increase the patient's well-being toward a higher level (Pender, Murdaugh, & Parsons, 2002).

The health promotion model proposes that each individual is unique, with a special set of experiences and characteristics that influence his or her actions. The specific variables related to behavior are important in terms of motivational factors for each individual. These variables can be affected by nursing actions and hopefully will positively influence health-promoting behavior. Health-promoting behavior on the part of the individual should result in an improved overall level of health and quality of life across the person's life span (Pender et al, 2002).

Like other theoretical models in nursing, the Pender health promotion model has specific assumptions and scientific proposals that provide both its unique properties and the boundaries that distinguish it as a model (Pender et al., 2002):

- The individual seeks to create living conditions that allow the expression of his or her unique health potential.
- The individual is capable of reflective self-awareness and is able to assess his or her own competency as a person.
- The individual values growth in a positive direction and tries to generate a balance between change and stability that is acceptable to him or her.
- The individual tries to regulate his or her own behavior as a person.
- The individual has biopsychosocial complexity, and because of this, he or she interacts with the environment and is constantly changing it and simultaneously being changed over time.
- The nurse makes up part of the interpersonal environment, and this influences the individual throughout the course of his or her life span.
- For behavior to change, the person must also change his or her pattern of interaction that occurs between that person and the environment.

The Pender model also has several *theoretical propositions*. These statements act as a foundation for research to be performed on health behaviors (Pender et al., 2002):

< The individual's beliefs, affect, and implementation of health-promoting behavior are influenced by prior behavior and characteristics that are either inherited or acquired.
< The individual will commit to engaging in a behavior if he or she believes a benefit can be derived from engaging in that behavior.
< The individual may fail to implement specific behaviors if barriers are perceived.
< The individual may choose to implement specific behaviors if he or she believes in the competence to carry out those behaviors.
< The more competent the individual believes he or she is, the fewer the barriers present and inhibiting specific health behaviors.
< Positive affect toward a proposed health behavior results in greater competence on the part of the individual, which in turn results in increased positive affect.
< The greater the level of positive emotions or affect associated with a proposed behavior, the greater the likelihood the individual will be committed to the behavior and will implement it.
< An individual is more likely to commit to and implement a health-promoting behavior when significant others model the behavior, anticipate the behavior occurring, and function as a support system to encourage implementation of the behavior.
< Family members, the individual's peer group, and healthcare providers can influence the individual's commitment to and complete engagement in health-promoting behaviors.
< Situations existing in the surrounding environment can increase or decrease the likelihood that the individual will or will not be committed to participating in the health-promoting behavior.
< Health-promoting behaviors are more likely to be maintained over a period of time if there is a significant commitment by the individual to a specific plan of implementation.
< When the individual who is committed to a plan for implementing health-promoting behavior has multiple demands that compete for his or her attention, there is decreased likelihood that the person will remain committed to the behavior.
< When the individual who is committed to a plan for implementation of health-promoting behavior has other actions available that are viewed

as preferable to the proposed behavior, commitment to the health-promoting behavior is likely to decrease.

< The individual can alter his or her thinking patterns, affect, support system, and surrounding environment to create incentives for implementation of health-promoting actions.

Whereas Pender's model explains the concept of health promotion and how an individual develops the commitment to implement behaviors to benefit his or her behavior, the transtheoretical model of change describes how an individual actually changes a problematic behavior.

Transtheoretical Model of Change

The *transtheoretical model of change* focuses on the decision-making ability of the individual to make an intentional change in his or her behavior. It proposes that a change in behavior is a process that occurs over time (Velicer, Prochaska, Fava, Norman, & Redding, 1998). The transtheoretical model of change proposes that a health-promoting modification in an individual's behavior occurs in a process of five separate stages (**Table 6-3**):

< *Precontemplation*: In this stage the individual does not intend to take action toward making a change in behavior for at least 6 months. The person may have already unsuccessfully attempted to change or may simply lack information about the consequences of his or her behavior and the subsequent need to change. At this stage the person does not want to discuss his or her behavior or consider the high-risk nature of choices being made. The person will frequently be perceived as unmotivated or resistant to the idea of a change in behavior.

< *Contemplation*: In this stage the individual has intentions of changing his or her behavior at some point in the next 6 months. He or she is equally aware of the advantages and disadvantages of changing his behavior. This awareness can promote ambivalence in the individual and can cause him or her to be labeled as a procrastinator.

< *Preparation*: In this stage the individual intends to take action within the next month. The person usually has some type of plan of action and functions well in an active form of behavioral change such as a weight loss program that relies heavily on exercise.

< *Action*: In this stage the individual has made obvious changes in his or her lifestyle within the past 6 months. The goal at this point is to reach a standard that health professionals have agreed on as being adequate to

TABLE 6-3 Stages of the Transtheoretical Model of Change

Stage	Description	Action of the Patient
Precontemplation	The individual does not intend to take action toward making a change in behavior for at least six months. The person may have already unsuccessfully attempted to change or may simply lack information about the consequences of their behavior and the subsequent need to change.	The person does not want to discuss his or her behavior or consider the high-risk nature of choices being made. The person will frequently are perceived as unmotivated or resistant to the idea of a change in behavior.
Contemplation	The individual has intentions of changing his or her behavior at some point in the next six months and is aware of the advantages and disadvantages of changing his behavior.	Awareness of the advantages and disadvantages of changing his behavior can promote ambivalence in the individual and can cause him or her to be labeled as a procrastinator.
Preparation	The individual intends to take action within the next month.	The person usually has some type of plan of action and functions well in an active form of behavioral change such as a weight loss program that relies heavily on exercise.
Action	The individual has made obvious changes in his or her lifestyle within the past six months.	The goal at this point is to reach a standard that health professionals have agreed upon as being adequate to sufficiently reduce the risk for disease and to prevent relapse.
Maintenance	The individual continues to work to prevent relapse.	The person has confidence that the change in behavior will continue.

Source: Velicer, W., Prochaska, J., Fava, J., Norman, G., & Redding, C., 1998.

sufficiently reduce the risk for disease. This stage is also crucial because of the monitoring to prevent relapse that must occur.

< *Maintenance*: In this stage the individual works to prevent relapse. The person has confidence the change in behavior will continue.

Thus far, Pender's health promotion model has explained how an individual develops the commitment to implement behaviors to benefit his or her health and the transtheoretical model of change has described how the person actually changes a problematic behavior that could have a negative effect on his or her health and quality of life. However, adoption of health-promoting behaviors will not occur without the individual's belief that his or her overall health and well-being will be enhanced through the integration of these behaviors. The health belief model attempts to explain how this will occur and to predict who will actually become fully engaged in health-promoting activities such as health screenings and immunizations against virulent diseases.

Health Belief Model

The *health belief model* proposes several primary perceptions that influence an individual's decision to take action to prevent illness (D'Amico & Barbarito, 2007) (**Table 6-4**):

< The person is potentially vulnerable to developing an illness: This is *perceived susceptibility* to illness. This can be visualized as a spectrum consisting of, on one end, individuals who completely deny any possibility of acquiring the disease. In the middle part of the spectrum are patients who recognize the possibility of acquiring the disease but believe such a situation is unlikely to affect them. At the opposite end of the spectrum are individuals who are so fearful of acquiring the disease they believe that in all likelihood they will develop it. The greater the level of susceptibility felt by an individual, the greater the likelihood that he or she will take preventive measures to avoid developing a specific disease process. The more susceptible a person feels, the greater the likelihood of his or her taking preventive measures.

< The effects of developing such an illness would be serious: This is the perceived severity of the potential illness. This can vary significantly from person to person and may consist of the person viewing the disease primarily from a

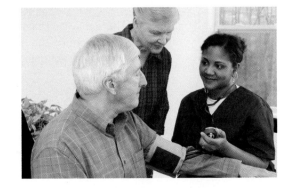

TABLE 6-4 Concepts of the Health Belief Model

Concept	Description	Action of the Individual
Perceived susceptibility	The person believes he or she is potentially vulnerable to developing an illness.	The greater the level of susceptibility felt by an individual, the greater the likelihood that he or she will take preventive measures to avoid developing a specific disease process. The more susceptible a person feels, the greater the likelihood of his or her taking preventive measures.
Perceived threat	The effects of developing such as illness would be serious.	This can vary significantly from person to person and may consist of the person viewing the disease primarily from a medical perspective and being concerned primarily with symptoms, potential for disability, and rate of mortality, while another person may view the disease in terms of the effect that the disease could have on his or her family members and ability to carry out job responsibilities.
Perceived benefits	There are advantages to use of the methods proposed for reducing the possibility of contracting the disease or reducing the seriousness of the illness resulting from the disease process promoting actions.	The perceived benefits of the health promoting action are greatly affected by the patient's knowledge of available alternatives for him or her.
Perceived barriers	There may be costs involved in implementing the new health-promoting actions.	Although a new action may reduce likelihood of contracting a specific disease process, implementing the action may prove to be costly, whether in terms of actual funds, or discomfort, or convenience.

Concept	Description	Action of the Individual
Cues to action	The person feels the need to take action to protect his or her health.	These cues are considered to be anything that motivates the person to take action to begin incorporating health-promoting behaviors. The cues can be internal if the person notices a symptom that motivates him or her to seek medical care, or external if the person reads an article that motivates him or her to make an appointment with a physician.
Self-efficacy	The person believes that he or she is capable of implementing a new health-promoting behavior.	This is the individual's confidence that he or she has the ability to incorporate a new behavior that will enhance his or her health.

Source: D'Amico & Barbarito, 2007.

medical perspective and being concerned primarily with symptoms, potential for disability, and rate of mortality, whereas another person may view the disease in terms of the effect the disease could have on his or her family members and his or her ability to carry out job responsibilities. Some experts combine the perceived susceptibility and perceived severity into *perceived threat*.

< There are advantages to use of the methods proposed for reducing the possibility of contracting the disease or reducing the seriousness of the illness resulting from the disease process: This is the *perceived benefit* to adoption of health-promoting actions, and it can be greatly affected by the patient's knowledge of available alternatives for him or her.

< There may be costs involved in implementing the new health-promoting actions: These are the *perceived barriers* and refer to the person's belief that although a new action may reduce likelihood of contracting a specific disease process, implementing the action may prove to be costly, whether in terms of actual funds, discomfort, or convenience.

< The person feels the need to take action to protect his or her health: This is known as the *cues to action*, and these cues are considered to be

anything that motivates the person to take action to begin incorporating health-promoting behaviors. The cues to action can be internal if the person notices a symptom that motivates him or her to seek medical care or external if the person reads an article that motivates him or her to make an appointment with a physician.

< The person believes he or she is capable of implementing a new health-promoting behavior: This is *self-efficacy* and refers to the individual's confidence that he or she has the ability to incorporate a new behavior to enhance his or her health.

Once there is sufficient understanding of models that explain how the process of health promotion takes place, how the patient's health beliefs affect his or her integration of health promotional behaviors, and how the process of integration of new beliefs occurs, activities that can promote health in a patient can be discussed.

Health Promotion Programs

Most health promotion programs include some type of information dissemination because an individual must have an adequate knowledge base to recognize a problem with his or her health status is present and there are alternatives for change available to the patient. Information dissemination can occur at the individual, group, or community level. Dissemination at the individual level can include the teaching performed before the discharge of a client from the hospital, whereas dissemination at the group level occurs when a class on managing the side effects of chemotherapy is offered to cancer patients at an oncologist's office. Dissemination at the community level can include use of an Internet discussion board on medical issues that is open to anyone that posts a comment (Wilkinson & Treas, 2011).

Health Promotion During the History and Physical

Heath promotion using primary prevention and both screening and counseling activities begins during the health history of the patient as well as during the review of body systems and the physical examination. The patient should be asked about family history of specific disease processes and the cause of death of various family members. If the patient cannot provide the information, obtain the information from the designated caregiver. The extent of the detail of the physical examination depends on the health history. The physical exam should include at the very least:

< Assessment of vital signs
< Weight
< Body mass index
< Waist circumference (can be used as an alternative to the body mass index)
< Auscultation and palpation of the chest and abdomen
< Inspection of the skin
< Palpation of peripheral pulses

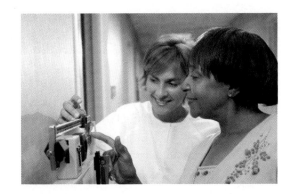

If at all possible, lab work should be done at the time of the physical examination so baseline levels of complete metabolic and lipid panels, thyroid function panel, and urinalysis can be obtained. Other lab work may be performed depending on the physical condition of the patient (Wilkinson & Treas, 2011).

Health Promotion During the Physical Fitness Assessment

The overall fitness of the individual should be determined along with a detailed history and completion of a physical examination. Regular physical exercise is known to be a health-promoting activity because of its association with a decreased risk for the development of cardiac disease, stroke, diabetes mellitus, hypertension, and other debilitating or potentially fatal illnesses. Regular physical exercise is particularly beneficial for the aging patient because it prevents excessive weight gain, improves muscle tone and bone density, and promotes improved cognitive abilities (Wilkinson & Treas, 2011).

An assessment of the patient's physical fitness should include the following (**Table 6-5**):

< Assessment of cardiopulmonary fitness: Demonstrated by the ability to perform large-muscle, moderate-to-high-intensity exercise for lengthy periods of time, such as would occur by the patient using a treadmill or stationary bicycle.
< Muscular fitness: Demonstrated by both muscle strength and degree of endurance. Muscle strength is considered to be a measure of the amount of weight a specific muscle group can move at any particular time, whereas muscle endurance is defined as the ability of a muscle to perform repetitive movements.

TABLE 6-5 **History and Physical Examination/Physical Fitness Assessment**

History	
Measure of Assessment	**Description**
Family history of specific disease processes	Health history will determine the extent of the detail of the health history
Cause of death of family members	Health history will determine the extent of the detail of the health history
Physical Assessment	
Assessment of vital signs, weight, body mass index, waist circumference (can be used as an alternative to the body mass index), auscultation and palpation of the chest and abdomen, inspection of the skin and palpation of peripheral pulses	Considered to be the minimum level of physical assessment performed
Lipid panel, thyroid function panel, and urinalysis	Need baseline levels of complete metabolic panel
Other types of labwork	Specific to the physical condition of the patient
Physical Fitness	
Assessment of cardiopulmonary fitness	Demonstrated by the ability to perform large-muscle, moderate-to-high-intensity exercise for lengthy periods of time, such as would occur with having the patient utilize a treadmill or stationary bicycle.
Assessment of muscular fitness	Demonstrated by both muscle strength and degree of endurance. Muscle strength is considered to be a measure of the amount of weight that a specific muscle group can move at any particular time, while muscle endurance is defined as the ability of a muscle to perform repetitive movements.
Assessment of flexibility	Demonstrated by the ability to move a joint through its entire range of motion, and is most frequently used to assess lower back and hip flexion.

Source: Wilkinson & Treas, 2011.

< Flexibility: Demonstrated by the ability to move a joint through its entire range of motion and is most frequently used to assess lower back and hip flexion (Wilkinson & Treas, 2011).

Lifestyle and Risk Appraisal

Lifestyle and risk appraisal encompass the manner in which the person conducts him- or herself in every facet of life, whether physical, emotional, spiritual, or mental. The person's lifestyle includes his or her occupation, recreational activities, and personal habits such as hobbies and can be defined as anything that promotes the highest quality of life for the patient. In addition, a *health risk appraisal* should be completed for the patient. This questionnaire evaluates the patient's risk for development of disease based on his or her current demographics, lifestyle, and current health-related practices. The health risk appraisal together with the lifestyle assessment provides a snapshot of the patient's view of health-promoting practices as well as risky practices and what he or she believes will ultimately provide the highest quality of life (Wilkinson & Treas, 2011).

Life Stress Review

Research has shown that prolonged exposure to stress can contribute significantly to the development of various forms of illness. In the 1920s Hans Selye first began to collect data on what would be the basis for his later published work on the stress response. He proposed that certain changes occur within the body of a patient subjected to prolonged stress that disrupt the normal physiological functioning of the body and ultimately trigger various disease processes (Selye, 1978). He referred to these changes as the *general adaptation syndrome* and believed that it consisted of three stages (**Table 6-6**):

< Alarm reaction: Any physical or mental trauma triggers a set of reactions in an attempt to respond to the stress. The immune system is initially depressed, levels of resistance are lowered, and the person becomes more vulnerable to development of disease. If the stress is short-lived, the individual bounces back and sustains a rapid recovery.
< Resistance: The individual adapts to stress and becomes more resistant to illness as the immune system works harder to accommodate the demands placed on it. The person assumes he or she is resistant to the effects of stress indefinitely and fails to take action to relieve the source of the stress.
< Exhaustion: The person sustains a sudden drop in his or her resistance level due to the body's inability to maintain homeostasis and the body

TABLE 6-6 Stages of the General Adaptation Syndrome

Stage of General Adaptation Syndrome	Description
Alarm	This consists of any physical or mental trauma that triggers a set of reactions in an attempt to respond to the stress. The immune system is initially depressed, levels of resistance are lowered, and the person becomes more vulnerable to development of disease. If the stress is short-lived, the individual bounces back and sustains a rapid recovery.
Resistance	The individual adapts to stress and becomes more resistant to illness as the immune system works harder to accommodate the demands placed upon it. The person assumes that he or she is resistant to the effects of stress indefinitely, and fails to take action to relieve the source of the stress.
Exhaustion	The person sustains a sudden drop in his or her resistance level due to the body's inability to maintain homeostasis and the body becomes susceptible to various disease processes.

Source: Selye, 1978.

becomes susceptible to various disease processes (Leyden-Rubenstein, 1999).

In modern society stressors that occur on a daily basis can include work-related deadlines, integrating blended families, and even the tension generated by the unstable economy. However, Judkins, Reid, and Furlow (2006) noted that such daily immersion into stress can be buffered by a characteristic known as hardiness (**Table 6-7**). First discussed by Kobasa, (Leyden-Rubenstein, 1999) individuals who possess hardiness are known to withstand pressure, succumb to stress-related illness less often, and adapt to persistent degrees of stress.

Hardiness is a set of beliefs held by the individual about him- or herself and the world; it is a valuable tool because it changes the way in which the individual views stress and it also makes available coping strategies to deal with the degree of stress experienced. The individual who possesses hardiness believes that factors creating stress can be changed and that he or she can therefore influence what occurs in the environment to produce stress. Hardiness is made up of three factors: control, commitment, and challenge. Hardy individuals

TABLE 6-7 Characteristics of Hardiness	
Characteristic	**Description**
Control	The individual has a high degree of control because he believes that he can influence the level of stress that he is experiencing and thus can change the factors producing it.
Commitment	The individual is immersed in the activities of life, believes what he does is both interesting and important, and actively engages in problem-solving to improve the work environment for all employees, not only himself.
Challenge	The individual believes that change is positive and thus is challenged by stressful situations and daily disruptions because they cause him or her to grow as a person and develop new coping strategies.

have a high degree of *control* because they believe they can influence the level of stress experienced and thus can change the factors producing it. Furthermore, the individual is immersed in the activities of life, believes what he or she does is both interesting and important, and actively engages in problem solving to improve the work environment for all employees, not only him- or herself. This is his or her degree of *commitment*. Finally, the hardy individual believes change is positive and thus is *challenged* by stressful situations and daily disruptions because they cause him or her to grow as a person and to develop new coping strategies. Such a person clearly understands the concept of health promotion and demonstrates primary prevention throughout his or her daily life (Judkins et al., 2006).

Summary of Key Points in Chapter

The chapter focused on aspects of health promotion. In addition to discussing health promotion as a concept and the types of health promotion, the chapter described the following:

< The primary, secondary, and tertiary levels of disease prevention along with examples of how these areas could be used in nursing practice.

‹ Models that pertain to health promotion, including Pender's model of health promotion, the transtheoretical model of change, and the health belief model, and a discussion of how these models describe the process that occurs when a patient decides to incorporate health-promoting action into his or her life.

‹ Programs in nursing practice that incorporate health promotion, including patient histories, physical examinations, physical fitness assessments, assessment of patient lifestyle, assessment of patient risk appraisal, and life stress review

Conclusion

As the American population's life span continues to widen, we must be more vigilant to practice health promotion and all levels of disease prevention to ensure the quality of life is equal to the length of those years. However, with a lengthening life span also comes the question of when it is appropriate for a patient to die and what the nurse's role should be as a patient begins the dying process. Such issues along with other legal and ethical issues pertaining to the modern registered nurse are discussed in the next chapter.

Critical Thinking Questions

1. You are a registered nurse working for a health maintenance organization designing health promotion plans. You are working with a 58-year-old African American man who has a history of cigarette smoking, hypertension, diabetes mellitus, and obesity. Consider the different types of health promotion activities and design a plan for this client that will result in an accurate risk assessment as well as appropriate counseling.

2. Consider your current work environment. Can you think of a recent patient care situation that could have been resolved more effectively if the assumptions and theoretical propositions of Pender's model of health promotion had been applied to it? Describe the situation in detail, including how it was resolved. Also, describe how the situation might have been resolved differently with the application of Pender's assumptions and propositions.

3. Consider Pender's model of health promotion in relation to the other models of nursing theory discussed previously. Which models appear

to have influenced Pender in her development of the health promotion model? Be able to support your answer.

4. Consider your current work environment. Can you think of a recent patient care situation that could have been resolved more effectively if the stages of the transtheoretical model of change had been applied to it? Describe the situation in detail, including how it was resolved. Also, describe how the situation might have been resolved differently with the application of the concepts of the transtheoretical model of change.

5. Consider the transtheoretical model of change in relation to the other models of nursing theory discussed previously. Which nursing models appear to have influenced development of the transtheoretical model of change? Be able to support your answer.

6. Compare and contrast the basic concepts of Pender's health promotion model, the transtheoretical model of change, and the health belief model.

7. You are preparing to document a history and perform a physical examination on a patient who arrived at the health clinic complaining of midsternal chest pain. Describe the most important areas to include in a history and a physical examination of this patient that would be considered to be health promotional.

8. After documentation of a history and physical examination on a patient who has arrived at the health clinic complaining of midsternal chest pain, you are preparing to assess the patient's physical fitness. Describe the most important areas to include in a physical fitness examination of this patient that would be considered to be health promotional.

9. After documenting a history and physical examination and physical fitness assessment on a patient who has arrived at the health clinic complaining of midsternal chest pain, you are preparing to asses the patient's lifestyle and risk appraisal. Describe the most important areas to include in a lifestyle and risk appraisal of this patient that would be considered to be health promotional.

10. After documentation of a history and physical examination, physical fitness assessment, and lifestyle and risk appraisal assessment on a patient who has arrived at the health clinic complaining of midsternal chest pain, you are preparing to complete a life stress review. Describe the most important areas to include in a life stress review of this patient that would be considered to be health promotional.

Scenarios

1. You are a registered nurse working for a health maintenance organization designing health promotion plans. You are working with a 58-year-old African American man who has a history of cigarette smoking, hypertension, diabetes mellitus, and obesity. He had a minor stroke 3 months ago and now walks with a slight limp on his right side. Since that time he has also experienced depression. Design a set of primary prevention strategies for this patient along with the expected outcomes that you anticipate resulting from the strategies.

2. You are a registered nurse working for a health maintenance organization designing health promotion plans. You are working with a 58-year-old African American man who has a history of cigarette smoking, hypertension, diabetes mellitus, and obesity. He had a minor stroke 3 months ago and now walks with a slight limp on his right side. Since that time he has also experienced depression. Design a set of secondary prevention strategies for this patient along with the expected outcomes that you anticipate resulting from the strategies.

3. You are a registered nurse working for a health maintenance organization designing health promotion plans. You are working with a 58-year-old African American man who has a history of cigarette smoking, hypertension, diabetes mellitus, and obesity. He had a minor stroke 3 months ago and now walks with a slight limp on his right side. Since that time he has also experienced depression. Design a set of tertiary prevention strategies for this patient along with the expected outcomes that you anticipate resulting from the strategies.

4. You are working with a patient who is a newly diagnosed diabetic. She is a 55-year-old legal secretary who is 5′3″ tall and weighs 185 pounds according to the scales in your office. She tells you she also runs a catering business on the weekends and specializes in creating wedding cakes. The patient admits to failing to see her primary care provider for the past 5 years because of her anxiety over her weight gain. Upon examination of the patient you note decreased sensation in both of her feet and find that the fourth toe of each foot is reddened. Use Pender's model of health promotion to describe the variables affecting this patient as you instruct her regarding health promotional behaviors.

5. Consider the patient described in scenario 4. Use the transtheoretical model of change to describe the process that will occur as this patient attempts to change her behaviors to more health-promoting actions.

6. Consider the patient described in scenario 4. Use the health belief model to describe the perceptions and cues to action affecting the patient as she attempts to adopt new health-promoting behaviors.

7. You have been put in charge of a task force that aims to increase public awareness of a particular genetic syndrome because there is an increased incidence of the disease in your community. Design a way to disseminate information about the disease at the individual, group, and community levels.

8. Consider the characteristics of hardiness: control, commitment, and challenge. Based on these characteristics, do you believe you possess hardiness as an individual? Why or why not? Be able to support your answer.

NCLEX® Questions

Using the information you obtained from studying this chapter, go online to complete the following NCLEX®-format review questions. Visit http://go.jblearning.com/terryLPN using the access code in the front cover of your book. This interactive resource allows you to answer each question and instantly review your results. Practice until you can answer at least 75% successfully, and then try to improve your score with each successive attempt.

Match the descriptor with the appropriate model.

1. precontemplation
2. perceived susceptibility
3. alarm reaction
4. self-efficacy
5. resistance
6. reflective self awareness
7. perceived barrier
8. preparation
9. exhaustion
10. biopsychosocial complexity
11. cues to action
12. contemplation
13. change-stability balance
14. behavioral self-regulation
15. perceived threat

16. action
17. behavioral commitment
18. positive growth
19. perceived benefit
20. maintenance
     a. Pender's model of health promotion
     b. transtheoretical model of change
     c. health belief model
     d. general adaptation syndrome

For more information on the topics in this chapter and others, please see Appendix on p. 299 for a list of web links to additional resources.

References

D'Amico, D., & Barbarito, C. (2007). *Health and physical assessment in nursing.* Upper Saddle River, NJ: Pearson.

Finkelman, A. (2012). *Leadership and management for nurses* (2nd ed.). Boston, MA: Pearson.

Irmak, Z., & Fesci, H. (2010). Effects of nurse-managed secondary prevention program on lifestyle and risk factors of patients who had experienced myocardial infarction. *Applied Nursing Research, 23,* 147–152.

Judkins, S., Reid, B., & Furlow, L. (2006). Hardiness training among nurse managers: Building a healthy workplace. *Journal of Continuing Education in Nursing, 37,* 202–207.

Leyden-Rubenstein, L. (1999). *The Stress Management Handbook: Strategies for Health and Inner Peace.* New Canaan, CT: Keat Publishing.

Mahon, S. (2005). Tertiary prevention: Implications for improving the quality of life of long-term survivors of cancer. *Seminars in Oncology Nursing, 21,* 260–270.

Pender, N., Murdaugh, C., & Parsons, M. (2002). *Health promotion in nursing practice* (4th ed.). Upper Saddle River, NJ: Prentice-Hall.

Selye, H. (1978). *The Stress of Life.* New York, NY: McGraw-Hill.

U.S. Department of Health and Human Services. (2010). *HHS announces the nation's new health promotion and disease prevention agenda.* Retrieved from http://www.healthypeople.gov/2020/about/DefaultPressRelease.pdf

Velicer, W., Prochaska, J., Fava, J., Norman, G., & Redding, C. (1998). Smoking cessation and stress management: Applications of the Transtheoretical Model of behavior change. *Homeostasis, 38,* 216–233.

Wilkinson, J., & Treas, L. (2011). *Fundamentals of nursing* (2nd ed.). Philadelphia, PA: F.A. Davis.

Williams, H. (2008). Primary prevention in health promotion. *The Pulse.* Retrieved from http://findarticles.com/p/articles/mi_6876/is_2_45/ai_n28548304/.

For a full suite of assignments and additional learning activities, use the access code located in the front of your book to visit this exclusive website: http://go.jblearning.com/terryLPN. If you do not have an access code, you can obtain one at the site.

www

At the end of this chapter, you will be able to:

1. Compare and contrast major aspects of public law and civil law.

2. Describe the significance of the Nurse Practice Act to the registered nurse.

3. Discuss ethical dilemmas that may face the registered nurse in modern health care.

4. Describe the significance of the American Nurses Association code of ethics to the registered nurse.

5. Discuss the various types of torts that can affect the nurse's practice.

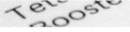

KEY TERMS

www

administrative law

advanced directives

alcohol/substance abuse by a nurse

American Nurses Association code of ethics

assault

autonomy

battery

beneficence

civil law

confidentiality

constitutional law

contract law

criminal conviction of a nurse

criminal law

"do not resuscitate" orders

due process

durable power of attorney

encrypted

ethical dilemma

euthanasia

fidelity

futile care

Health Insurance Portability and Accountability Act

justice

living will

malpractice

moral courage

moral distress

multistate licensure compact

negligence

nonmaleficence

Nurse Practice Act

Patient Self-Determination Act

privacy

public law

role conflict

tort

unethical/unprofessional practice by a nurse

unprofessional conduct by a nurse

unsafe practice by a nurse

veracity

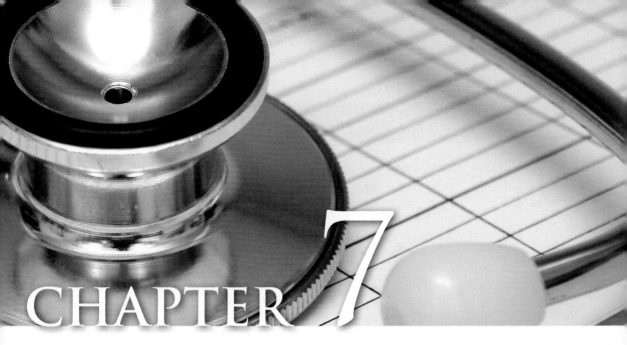

CHAPTER 7

Legal–Ethical Aspects of Nursing

Introduction to Legal–Ethical Aspects of Nursing

As the licensed practical nurse moves into the role of registered nurse (RN), the transition will involve successfully completing the NCLEX-RN®. This step is necessary to provide the new RN with a license to practice nursing in his or her state of choice and subsequently to give the new practitioner a legal status affected by various types of law. Here we discuss the types of law that affect the RN, including the type that provides his or her initial licensure to practice.

Although the constitution is the set of laws that grants the authority to make, implement, and interpret laws, it falls to the state and federal legislative bodies to enact these laws. Major sources of law that affect nursing practice are public law and civil law.

Public Law

Public law includes constitutional law, criminal law, and administrative law (Kelly, 2010) (**Table 7-1**). *Constitutional law* refers to a citizen's rights, privileges, and responsibilities provided through the Constitution of the United States, including those documented in the Bill of Rights. States are not allowed to pass laws that conflict with these rights because the Constitution is considered to be the highest source of American law (Zerwekh & Garneau, 2012).

TABLE 7-1 Types of Public Law

Type of Law	Description	Effect on Nurses
Constitutional law	Refers to a citizen's rights, privileges, and responsibilities that are provided through the U.S. Constitution, including those documented in the Bill of Rights. States are not allowed to pass laws that conflict with these rights because the Constitution is considered to be the highest source of American law.	The nurse cannot violate a patient's rights to 1. Freedom of Speech, Press, Religion, and Petition 2. Right to Keep and Bear Arms 3. Conditions for Quarters of Soldiers 4. Search and Seizure Regulated 5. Provisions Concerning Prosecution 6. Right to a Speedy Trial, Witnesses, etc. 7. Right to Trial by Jury 8. Excessive Bail, Cruel Punishment Prevented 9. Rule of Construction of Constitution 10. Rights of the States Under the Constitution
Criminal law	Refers to actions of individuals that are intentionally directed to harm members of the public.	Nurses are affected because of the mandate to protect vulnerable populations of patients. Most states require nurses to report suspected abuse of children or older adults. Failure to report such acts can result in severe penalties for the nurse. Criminal law also affects nurses and their practice through the use of criminal background checks. Potential employees who would be working with children or older adults are required to have criminal background checks. Failure of a facility to implement this can result in monetary loss if an employee who did not receive a background check later causes harm to a patient. It is the nurse's responsibility as the potential employee to provide accurate and truthful information. If the nurse is the authority supervising the procedure of implementing background checks, it is his or her responsibility to ensure that the procedure is carried out for every prospective employee.

Type of Law	Description	Effect on Nurses
		Criminal law can affect the nurse and his or her practice through the stipulation that the health professional licensed to practice nursing cannot engage in substance abuse. Although employing facilities can implement random drug screens of employees at any time, a nurse's employment can also be affected by use of drugs and alcohol outside of the workplace. If a nurse is found to be abusing drugs and/or alcohol outside of the work setting, the nurse may have employment terminated and his or her license either disciplined or revoked by the employing state's Board of Nursing.
Administrative law	This type of law deals with protecting the rights of citizens.	In the federal system, the Occupational Safety and Health Administration develops regulations that will affect healthcare workers, including how hazardous substances will be stored, procedures to protect employees from infectious substances, and policies to protect employees from falling victim to workplace violence.

Source: Zerwekh & Garneau, 2012; Kelly, 2010.

Criminal law refers to actions of individuals that are intentionally directed to harm members of the public. Nurses are specifically affected by this area of law because of the mandate to protect vulnerable populations of patients. Most states require nurses to report suspected abuse of children or older adults. Failure to report such heinous acts can result in severe penalties for the health professional (Kelly, 2010).

Criminal law also affects nurses and their practice through the use of criminal background checks. Certain categories of potential employees who will work with either children or older adults, such as in daycare settings or long-term care facilities, are required to have criminal background checks. Failure of a facility to implement such a requirement can result in substantial monetary loss if an employee who did not receive a background check later causes harm to a patient. It is the nurse's responsibility as the potential employee to pro-

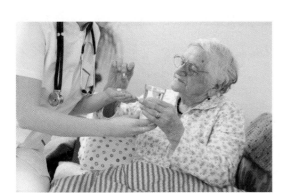

vide accurate and truthful information to expedite the procedure. The nurse in charge of implementing background checks is responsible for ensuring the procedure is carried out thoroughly and accurately and that no prospective employee is omitted from having such a check implemented (Kelly, 2010).

In addition, criminal law can affect the nurse and his or her practice through the stipulation that the health professional who is licensed to practice nursing cannot engage in substance abuse. Healthcare agencies that use regulated narcotic medications with their patient populations are required by both state and federal law to keep an accurate count of how these medications are used. Nurses are frequently called on to sign a record noting the issuing of a narcotic medication to a specific patient or to serve as a witness that a partial dose of medication that was not used was destroyed. Although employing facilities can implement random drug screens of employees at any time, a nurses' employment can also be affected by use of drugs and alcohol outside of the workplace. A nurse found to be abusing drugs and/or alcohol outside of the work setting may have employment terminated and his or her license either disciplined or revoked by the employing state's board of nursing (Kelly, 2010).

Finally, *administrative law* deals with protecting the rights of citizens. In the federal system the Occupational Safety and Health Administration develops regulations that affect healthcare workers, including how hazardous substances will be stored, procedures to protect employees from infectious substances, and policies to protect employees from falling victim to workplace violence (Kelly, 2010).

Another very important part of administrative law is each state's Nurse Practice Act. Each state's *Nurse Practice Act* gives that state's board of nursing the authority to define

‹ How nursing will be practiced in that locale
‹ Educational preparation required to practice as either a licensed practical/vocational nurse or registered nurse in that state
‹ How professional nurses will be disciplined if they do not adhere to the rules governing nursing practice

In addition, each state's board of nursing determines if that state will agree to recognize nursing licenses from other states, such as occurs through the multistate licensure compact. The *multistate licensure compact* allows an agreement to be developed between specific states to enable nurses licensed in one state to practice in another state without being required to apply for a new license. However, as of 2011 only 24 states have opted to participate in the multistate licensure compact, thus indicating the level of concern centered on this area of administrative law (Smith, 2009).

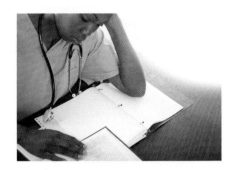

Nurse Practice Act

Each state's board of nursing is charged with investigating complaints brought against a nurse by the public to determine if the evidence is sufficient to bring discipline against the nurse's license. Some of the most common reasons for discipline being brought against a nurse's license follow (Smith, 2009) (**Table 7-2**):

< *Unprofessional conduct by a nurse*: Conduct that is likely to deceive or harm the public, such as would occur when a person uses false documentation to obtain a nursing license.

< *Unsafe practice by a nurse*: Negligence occurs in care delivery, resulting in delivery of incompetent care. State boards of nursing will initiate disciplinary actions against nurses for malpractice as well as negligence in practice. Criminal action can also be brought against the nurse if state attorneys choose to intervene in such an area.

< *Unethical and unprofessional practice of a nurse*: This area can include breach of patient confidentiality; engaging in sexual relations with patients; initiating sexual harassment of patients or staff members; and discriminating against a patient based on his or her ethnicity, religion, or other significant characteristics.

< *Criminal convictions of a nurse*: Nurses can receive discipline from their state boards of nursing if they receive criminal convictions, are convicted of a felony, or are convicted of any type of crime involving gross immorality. This can include fraud, misrepresentation, embezzlement of funds, patient abuse, and murder. Some states' boards of nursing have opted to prevent such nurses from practicing nursing for several years after a conviction.

< *Alcohol or substance abuse by a nurse*: Although discipline may occur, many boards are recognizing the need for the nurse who engages in substance abuse to undergo treatment in the hope of ultimately returning a competent practitioner back into the healthcare community. Some boards of nursing now encourage impaired nurses to report themselves

TABLE 7-2 Common Reasons for Discipline Being Brought Against a Nurse's License

Reason for Discipline	Description	Example
Unprofessional conduct	Conduct that is likely to deceive or harm the public	Using false documentation to obtain a nursing license
Unsafe practice	Negligence occurs in care delivery, resulting in delivery of incompetent care	Malpractice, negligence in practice
Unethical/ unprofessional practice	Conduct that violates the ANA Code of Ethics	This can include breach of patient confidentiality; engaging in sexual relations with patients; sexual harassment of patients or staff members; and discriminating against a patient based on ethnicity, religion, or other characteristic.
Criminal conviction	Nurses can receive discipline from their state's board of nursing if they receive criminal convictions, are convicted of a felony, or are convicted of any type of crime involving gross immorality.	This can include fraud, misrepresentation, embezzlement of funds, patient abuse, as well as murder.
Alcohol/substance abuse	In some states, discipline may be avoided if the nurse reports him/herself as using alcohol/ drugs and enters a treatment program.	Obvious evidence of alcohol or drug use

Source: Smith, 2009.

as engaging in substance abuse so they can enter a treatment facility and thus avoid discipline brought against their license.

Discipline of a Nurse's License

The ability of a state board of nursing to bring discipline against a nurse's license is based on the 14th Amendment to the Constitution. This amendment ensures no state can deprive someone of life, liberty, or property without due process of law. In the case of a nurse, there is property interest in the nursing

license because of its ability to ensure the nurse's liveli-
hood through the practice of nursing. *Due process* also
means that discipline of the nurse's license cannot occur
without following a previously established legal procedure. The board of nursing is required to notify the nurse
of the charges to be brought against him or her and the
basis of the charges. In addition, the nurse has a right to
a hearing in which he or she will be able to hear the evidence against him or her, to question witnesses, and also
to produce evidence and witnesses (Smith, 2009).

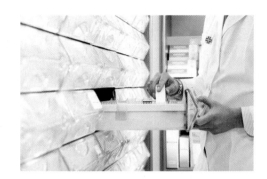

The process of bringing discipline against a nurse's license begins when
a member of the public brings a complaint against the nurse to the board of
nursing. Anyone can bring such a complaint to the attention of the board,
whether it is a patient who has undergone treatment at the hands of the nurse,
an employer who has noted an unsafe practice by the nurse, or a colleague
who has detected evidence of unprofessional conduct. The employer has an
obligation to report the following behaviors (Smith, 2009):

< Patient abandonment, such as may occur if the nurse accepts a patient
  assignment and then chooses to walk out of the facility
< Patient abuse, such as may occur if the nurse strikes a patient
< Patient neglect, such as may occur if the nurse does not take sufficient
  precautions to prevent a patient from falling
< Diversion of medications, such as may occur if a nurse takes a patient's
  narcotics for personal use

Once the complaint is received by the board of nursing, it is assigned to
an investigator who reviews the complaint and decides if it is of enough significance to warrant the collection of additional information. The investigator
then contacts the nurse, and an administrative hearing may be arranged. The
nurse has the option to have an attorney with him or her when talking with
the investigator. After the investigation is implemented, the board of nursing
makes a decision as to whether further action will be taken in the form of a
formal administrative hearing or whether to suspend the nurse's license. Immediate suspension may be implemented if the nurse is judged to be a danger
to the public (Smith, 2009).

Civil Law

In addition to public law, the nurse can be affected by civil law. *Civil law* refers to how individuals relate to each other in daily life and consists of both

contract law and tort law (**Table 7-3**). *Contract law* regulates certain types of transactions between individuals and businesses and between businesses. For an agreement to be recognized as a legal contract, it must contain the following points:

< Must be agreed on by two or more legally competent individuals or parties and must state what each party must or must not do
< Mutual understanding of the stipulations imposed on each party involved in the contract
< Some type of payment given in exchange for the actions that were taken or not taken as part of implementing the contract

The nurse can be affected by contract as an employee. The nurse who is employed agrees to adhere to the facility's policies and procedures, fulfills the duties of the employer that have already been agreed on by both parties, and

TABLE 7-3 Types of Civil Law

Type of Civil Law	Description	Effect on Nurses
Contract law	*Contract law* regulates certain types of transactions between individuals and businesses, as well as transactions between businesses. In order for an agreement to be recognized as a legal contract, it must be agreed upon by two or more legally competent individuals and must state what each party must or must not do to show mutual understanding of the stipulations that will be imposed on each party involved in the contract, and must show some type of payment given in exchange for the actions that were taken or not taken as part of implementing the contract.	The nurse who is employed agrees to adhere to the facility's policies and procedures, fulfill the duties of the employer that have already been agree upon by both parties, and respect the rights and responsibilities of the other employees working in the facility. The employer agrees to pay the nurse a specific amount for services rendered, agrees to give the nurse adequate assistance in providing care, to provide the supplies and equipment needed to fulfill required responsibilities, and to provide reasonable treatment and behavior from the other healthcare providers who will be interacting with the nurse in the work environment.

Type of Civil Law	Description	Effect on Nurses
Tort law	A *tort* is a negligent or intentional wrong not connected with a contract that injures a person, and for which the injured party may opt to sue the responsible person for damages. Torts commonly include denying a person his or her legal rights, failing to comply with public duties, and failing to perform a duty owed to a person that results in harm occurring to another person.	
	Assault consists of threatening to touch another person in a manner that is offensive to that person and without his or her permission.	
	Battery consists of actually carrying out the threat and touching the person without his permission.	
	Malpractice consists of a professional's wrongful conduct in carrying out his or her duties as a professional, leading to harm ensuing to another person entrusted to his or her care.	
	Negligence consists of failing to provide the care that a reasonable professional would provide in a similar situation.	
	If a nurse is charged with malpractice or negligence, damages can only be recovered if proof of fault on the part of the nurse can be proven. In order for fault to be proven, the following areas must be able to be shown: duty/obligation owed to the person by the nurse; a breach of this duty, whether intentionally or unintentionally; harm has been done to the injured party; and proof that the breach of duty caused the harm leading to initiation of the lawsuit.	

Source: Kelly, 2010.

respects the rights and responsibilities of the other employees working in the facility. In addition, the employer agrees to pay the nurse a specific amount for services rendered, to give the nurse adequate assistance in providing care, to provide the supplies and equipment needed to fulfill required responsibilities, and to provide reasonable treatment and behavior from the other healthcare providers who will be interacting with the nurse in the work environment (Kelly, 2010).

Another form of civil law is tort law. A *tort* is a negligent or intentional wrong not connected with a contract that injures a person and for which the injured party may opt to sue the responsible person for damages. Torts commonly include denying a person his or her legal rights, failing to comply with public duties, and failing to perform a duty owed to a person that results in harm occurring to another person. Torts can be intentional or unintentional.

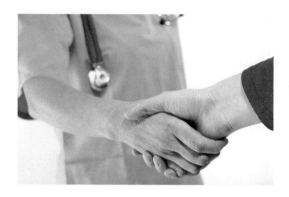

Examples of intentional torts are *assault* and *battery*. Assault consists of threatening to touch another person, such as a patient, in a manner that is offensive to that person and without his or her permission. Battery consists of actually carrying out the threat and proceeding to touch the person without having his or her permission. Examples of unintentional torts are *malpractice* or *negligence*. Malpractice consists of a professional's wrongful conduct in carrying out his or her duties as a professional, leading to harm ensuing to another person entrusted to his or her care. Negligence, in comparison, consists of failing to provide the care that a reasonable professional would provide in a similar situation. If a nurse is charged with malpractice or negligence, damages can only be recovered if fault on the part of the nurse can be proven. For fault to be proven, the following areas must be shown (Kelly, 2010):

<   A duty or obligation owed to the injured party by the nurse
<   A breach of this duty, whether intentionally or unintentionally
<   Harm has been done to the injured party
<   Breach of duty caused the harm leading to initiation of the lawsuit

Advanced Directives

The RN must have an understanding of how the concept of advanced directives affects the patient. An *advanced directive* is a set of instructions that give a person's wishes related to his or her health care if he or she were unable to make and verbalize a decision. Educating patients about advance directives is required by the *Patient Self-Determination Act*. This legislation also requires that patients be given the opportunity to complete an advance directive if so desired (Wilkinson & Treas, 2011).

There are two types of advance directives the RN may be required to discuss with a patient: the living will and the durable power of attorney. The *living will* is a document prepared by a competent person that gives instructions about the medical care that should be provided for that person if he or she becomes unable to make and verbalize decisions. Also specified are the types of health care a person would not want at the end of his or her life, such as specifying that he or she does not want to receive tube feedings. In comparison, the *durable power of attorney* exists when a competent person names another person to make decisions about his or her health care when unable to do so. The document frequently gives specific instructions about feeding tubes, cardiopulmonary resuscitation, and being placed on ventilators. Such a document must be witnessed by two people (Wilkinson & Treas, 2011).

Issues Involving Confidentiality

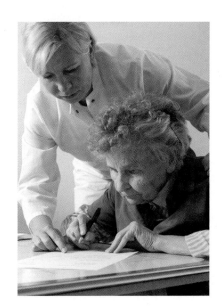

All patient information must be kept private and confidential. The *Health Insurance Portability and Accountability Act* (HIPAA) first brought privacy issues involving medical information to the public's attention in 1996. The legislation includes a system for ensuring privacy regarding health information that could potentially be used to identify a specific patient. Information used to provide treatment, payment, or any type of healthcare operation does not require a patient's specific consent for it to be used. This means a patient can be billed for a surgical procedure without having to give consent for "surgical procedure" to be typed onto the remittance slip. However, disclosure of any type of medical information must be at the bare minimum amount, only what is absolutely necessary. The patient must be notified of how the information will be used (Zerwekh & Garneau, 2012).

Additional requirements were added to HIPAA in 2005. These stipulated that to ensure that protected patient information is disclosed only on a "need to know basis," each institution must conduct its own risk assessment and develop data security policies and technologies in response to the assessment. The facility may opt to have information coded or *encrypted* when it is e-mailed over the Internet to ensure it is not accessed by someone who does not have a right to view it (Zerwekh & Garneau, 2012).

To ensure continuity of care for patients continues despite the HIPAA requirements, some states have enacted legislation to protect communication that occurs between healthcare providers and patients. This means that information can be communicated freely between physicians and patients without fear of it falling into the wrong person's access. Usually such a privilege is extended to nurses as well as physicians. Ultimately, though, it is the RN's responsibility to maintain confidentiality any time he or she has access to patient information. Such sensitive information should not be discussed with coworkers in the elevator where the public could overhear it or at home with the nurse's family members. Maintaining such a practice cannot only help avoid a lawsuit for the RN but can also allow the nurse to serve as a mentor and a role model for new graduate nurses as well (Zerwekh & Garneau, 2012).

Ethical Issues in Nursing

Ethical issues in the nursing profession can frequently be intertwined with legal issues as well. "Ethics in nursing" is a somewhat nebulous term but essentially refers to morals and values used when healthcare professionals make life-and-death decisions involving patients and their care. Healthcare professionals, and nurses in particular, frequently are faced with an *ethical dilemma*—a situation in which there seem to be a conflict between

< Two separate ethical duties owed to the patient
< The patient's rights and the benefits that he or she could expect
< A duty owed to the nurse and a duty owed to the patient
< Professional ethical requirements and religious beliefs of the nurse (Huber, 2010)

The RN faced with the existence of an ethical dilemma should first ensure he or she has a sufficient understanding of important ethical principles:

< *Autonomy*: This is the patient's right to make his or her own decisions
< *Beneficence*: This means the nurse wants to do good for the patient and balances the potential benefit to the patient with the potential risk
< *Nonmaleficence*: This means avoiding doing harm to the patient
< *Justice*: This equates to providing fair and equal treatment to all patients and to ensuring that benefits, risks, and costs are equally distributed so that no one group or individual bears the burden exclusively
< *Fidelity*: Pertains to being loyal to commitments that have been made and accountable for responsibilities
< *Veracity*: Pertains to avoiding misleading patients
< *Confidentiality*: Pertains to the amount of information that can be disclosed about a patient without his or her consent
< *Privacy*: Pertains to limiting the amount of information to disclose about oneself

These principles pertaining to ethics (**Table 7-4**) must be well understood by the RN before an ethical dilemma develops so that valuable time is not spent in lengthy deliberation (Huber, 2010).

ANA Code of Ethics

In addition to a clear understanding of the principles that form the foundation of nursing ethics, the RN should also adhere to the *American Nurses Association's* (ANA) *code of ethics*, a document containing the ethical

TABLE 7-4 Ethical Principles Used in Nursing

Ethical Principle	Description	Significance to RNs
Autonomy	Patient has the right to make his/her own decision	The RN helps the patient understand the nature and extent of his disease process and the possible outcomes of treatment. This will enable the patient to make the best possible decision about his health care based on all available information.
Beneficence	The nurse wants to do good for the patient; the potential benefit to the patient is weighed against the potential risk	The RN will provide the patient with the information that will help him reduce risk of harm by making choices based on all available information.
Nonmaleficence	Avoiding doing harm to the patient	The RN will make every effort to protect the well-being of the patient and will not allow actions that could cause harm to the patient.
Justice	Fair and equitable treatment to all patients	The RN must treat all people fairly without considering socioeconomic status, personal characteristics, or the basis for the patient's health problems.
Fidelity	Being loyal to commitments and accountable for responsibilities	The RN will stay faithful to the nurse–patient relationship that has been forged with the patient.
Veracity	Avoiding misleading patients	The RN provides the patient with truthful information; this will allow the patient to make evidence-based decisions about his health care.
Confidentiality	Pertains to the amount of information that can be disclosed about a patient without his/her consent	The RN will not allow protected health information to be released about the patient.
Privacy	Limiting the amount of information to disclose about oneself	The patient expects the RN to guard his privacy, and the RN protects him from harm that could result from a breach in his privacy.

Source: Huber, 2010.

obligations and duties of the nurse. The code does not provide specific answers for every ethical issue that could be faced by a nurse but instead provides general principles used to make decisions when the nurse is confronted with various types of ethical decisions. However, there are several areas of ethical uncertainty where the ANA code of ethics does provide more specific guidance to the RN (Huber, 2010):

‹ Patient's right to die
‹ Use of incentives to decrease spending in health care
‹ Confronted with questionable or impaired practice of a colleague
‹ Patient whose medical needs exceed the nurse's knowledge base and skill set
‹ Organization creating barriers to ethical practice

Ethical Decision-Making

How should the RN go about resolving an ethical dilemma when there seems to be a conflict between the professional duty owed to the patient, the rights of the patient, and possibly even the religious beliefs of the nurse? The basic problem-solving process can be modified to fit this situation (Huber, 2010):

‹ Define the problem by breaking it down into manageable terms. It may be easier to make a decision if the problem is broken down into a series of smaller problems that may be more easily solved.
‹ Determine the alternatives that are not only available but are truly options that are viable. If an alternative would only be feasible if there was additional equipment, personnel, and funding, it is not a true alternative.
‹ Evaluate all alternative courses of action, determining how easily each would be implemented, the resources that would be required, the benefits to all persons involved, and the drawbacks.
‹ Choose the best course of action based on weighing the benefits and the drawbacks.
‹ Implement the selected course of action, documenting every step of the process of implementation.
‹ Evaluate the results of the implementation process, monitoring it closely so as to provide guidance in the event that such an ethical dilemma occurs again.

Figure 7-1 shows the process of working through an ethical dilemma from start to finish.

FIGURE 7-1 **Process of Solving an Ethical Dilemma**

Determine that an ethical dilemma actually exists
(conflict between two ethical duties owed patient, patient's rights
and benefits expected, duty owed self and owed patient, or between
RN's professional ethical requirements and religious beliefs)

Develop a sufficient understanding of important ethical principles
(autonomy, beneficence, nonmaleficence, justice, fidelity,
veracity, confidentiality, privacy)

Define the problem
Determine alternatives available
Evaluate all alternatives available
Choose best course of action
Implement selected course of action
Evaluate results of implementation

Source: Huber, 2010.

Ethical Issues Related to Death and Dying

Multiple ethical dilemmas can emerge from the controversy that often surrounds the dying process and subsequent death. Frequently, nurses care for patients whose physicians have written *"do not resuscitate" orders*. These orders are enacted such that cardiopulmonary resuscitation is not used in the event the patient begins to exhibit signs that his or her physical condition is deteriorating. Such an order may be difficult for the nurse who believes that failing to resuscitate the patient is directly contributing to the patient's death and thus is in conflict with the nurse's duty to the patient (Rumbold, 1999).

For many RNs implementing such orders can create an ethical dilemma because of the nurse's concerns regarding *euthanasia*, the deliberate ending of life in the interest of ending the suffering of the patient. In addition, the nurse may have an ethical dilemma if called on to assist with a family's decision to withdraw life-sustaining treatment from a patient whose physical condition is deteriorating (Rumbold, 1999). This may conflict greatly with a nurse's commitment to sustain life as well as his or her religious beliefs regarding the sanctity of life.

Moral Distress

Ultimately, ethical dilemmas such as those just described can cause a nurse to experience *moral distress*, which Gallagher (2010) defined as the nurse knowing the right decision to make in a specific circumstance but being prevented from making the right decision by constraints imposed by the facility. Moral distress can be caused by a combination of substandard healthcare delivery; *futile care*, meaning care that seems to provide no benefit for the patient; unsuccessful advocacy by the RN on the behalf of the patient; and the belief that the RN is raising the patient's and family's hope unrealistically.

In the hospital work environment nurses report moral distress due to inadequate staffing as well as frequent confrontations with physicians. Research has shown that moral distress is associated with educational level and experience, suggesting nurses with advanced education and multiple years of experience tend to have higher levels of moral distress. It has been found to manifest itself physically in symptoms such as headaches, neck pain, and stomach problems and emotionally in the form of angry outbursts, feelings of guilt, frustration, low self-esteem, and isolation from loved ones. The main remedy for moral distress appears to be *moral courage*, which can be developed through the use of professional wisdom. The nurse who develops such wisdom typically is able to demonstrate the right response in the face of frightening encounters (Gallagher, 2010).

An RN should develop ways of knowing when moral distress is developing. Pendry (2007) noted several situations in the modern healthcare environment that can lead to the development of moral distress:

- *Role conflict*: This consists of the stress that develops when the expectations of two different areas of authority over a nurse are not congruent. For example, if the RN's hospital administration expects one thing from him or her and the physician that works closely with that nurse has a set of expectations that conflict with those of the hospital administration, role conflict results. Consequently, the RN will have more responsibility than authority and will lack the autonomy to accomplish what he or she believes needs to be done. The nurse will feel helpless and will believe that he or she is not able to provide high quality health care to patients.
- Conflict between physicians and nurses: Research has shown that the greatest conflict between physicians and nurses develops over end-of-life decision-making. Such conflicts can develop out of the multiple values that are involved, such as respect for human life as well as the patient's

right to autonomy, the hierarchy of authority present in most healthcare organizations, the lack of resources to devote to the patient in the midst of the dying process, and the need for all parties involved in the end-of-life decision-making process to have full communication with each other. Both physicians and nurses tend to express feelings of powerlessness in such a situation, with the physicians frequently expressing concern that selecting one patient to receive extended treatment might mean that another one receives a lesser degree of care, and nurses expressing concern that they are providing substandard care due to financial constraints. Research has shown that physicians typically feel the stress of making end-of-life decisions, whereas nurses feel the stress of implementing the mandates of a decision made by someone else.

< End-of-life care: Nurses frequently report being extremely stressed when patients ask for assistance in dying, particularly when they have been experiencing prolonged suffering. Nurses often express great concern over unrelieved pain and distress of patients as well as being asked to withhold nutrition or administer larger than recommended doses of opioid analgesics in an attempt to accelerate the dying process.

< Conflict between critical care and futile care: Critical care RNs are believed to experience particularly high levels of moral distress when called on to provide medically aggressive care to prolong life for a patient in a futile care situation, when clearly the patient is progressing into the dying process. It has been found that such a situation contributes significantly to the development of burnout in nurses, resulting in the RN experiencing emotional exhaustion, detachment, and a sense of lack of accomplishment. Moral distress can actually result from the critical care nurse's own expert judgment as a clinician because this sense will provide the nurse with a heightened perception of the inability to provide the patient with a prolonged quality of life.

< Managed care requirements: RNs who function under a managed care system have expressed moral distress as a result of the frustration over feeling they are functioning primarily as an agent for the health plan rather than as an advocate for the patient. Many nurses have reported feeling the need to exaggerate aspects of the patient's illness or purposely inadequately document patient findings to provide greater resources to the patient under the managed care system. RNs functioning as case managers have also reported moral distress resulting from the frustration in dealing with insurance companies. The case manager may be faced with attempting to advocate for the patient while trying to balance the dictates of the insurance company regarding how extensive care can be and the expectations of family members.

< Conflict between new graduates' expectations and reality: Research on the job satisfaction of new graduate nurses has shown that almost one-third of them report leaving their first nursing job within 1 year of being hired and more than half usually leave within 2 years. The new graduates who were surveyed reported they were greatly stressed by the acuity of the patients assigned to them, the nurse-to-patient ratios, their perceived inability to provide safe care, a lack of support and guidance, and a perception of having too much responsibility (Pendry, 2007).

Summary of Key Points in Chapter

Although this chapter discussed legal and ethical aspects of nursing, a wide variety of topics was presented. This included a discussion of the various types of public law (constitutional law, criminal law, and administrative law) and civil law (contract law and tort law). Under public law the importance of administrative law's creation of state boards of nursing was emphasized. The significance of the types of advance directives as well as HIPAA to the RN was reviewed.

Regarding ethics, the importance of the ANA code of ethics to the RN was discussed as well as the process for resolving an ethical dilemma. Finally, the characteristics of moral distress were delineated, as well various factors that could contribute to development of such a situation.

Conclusion

This chapter has shown multiple legal and ethical issues at work in the modern healthcare environment, and most of them will, at some point, have an effect on the RN and the care that he or she delivers. It is the responsibility of the RN who is transitioning into the process of becoming a nurse leader to stay up-to-the-minute with all available information on new developments in the legal arena that could affect not only his or her practice but the facility where that practice occurs. In addition, the RN nurse leader must maintain his or her status as a mentor and a role model in the healthcare community to recognize when other nurses are developing moral distress and to circumvent this process when possible.

Ethical issues such as those connected with the end of life are particularly stressful to deal with for the RN and could potentially result in legal difficulties as well. One concept that is closely related to the idea of ethical treatment of patients is that of how nursing care is affected by various cultural aspects of the patient. This idea is explored in the next chapter.

Critical Thinking Questions

1. Compare and contrast the major characteristics of constitutional, criminal, and administrative law.

2. Think about your own work environment and identify a situation that involved
   a. constitutional law
   b. criminal law
   c. administrative law

   How was each situation resolved? Do you believe any individual's rights were violated? At any point were patients endangered?

3. Compare and contrast the major points of contract law and tort law.

4. Describe how the RN can expect to be affected by
   a. constitutional law
   b. criminal law
   c. administrative law
   d. contract law
   e. tort law

5. Compare and contrast the major points of negligence and malpractice.

6. How can the RN expect to be affected by his or her state's Nurse Practice Act?

7. How would you explain the concepts of the living will and durable power of attorney to
   a. a physician who is undergoing surgery?
   b. a nurse who is undergoing surgery?
   c. a mechanic with an eighth grade education who is undergoing surgery?
   d. an immigrant who can speak and understand simple English but cannot read or write English?

8. Consider a current or past work environment. Can you recall a time when you saw a nurse exhibit moral distress? Have you ever felt moral distress? In addition, have you ever felt moral courage, or have you ever seen a nurse demonstrate it?

Scenarios

1. You are the nursing supervisor for a large hospital. While making rounds in the hospital one evening, you identify a nurse who appears to be intoxicated. What is the best action for you to implement at this time?

2. What is the best action for you to implement in 24 hours?

3. You are in charge of supervising the background check procedure for your hospital. You are notified that a prospective employee who is also a nurse has refused to submit to a background check. What is your best action at this time?

4. The nurse in scenario 3 agrees to submit to the background check but fails it. What is your best course of action now?

5. You are the director of nursing for a large hospital. You are notified that one of your employees, a nurse, failed a random urine drug test. What is your best course of action now?

6. What is your long-term plan for this employee?

7. You are the director of nursing for a large metropolitan hospital. You are informed that one of the nurses in the facility left the facility after being pulled to another floor to work for the day and accepting a patient assignment on that floor. What are the legal implications of this nurse's decision?

   a. What are the ethical implications of this nurse's decision?

   b. What should be your highest priority action as director of nursing after being informed of the situation?

8. You are the director of nursing of a large metropolitan hospital. You are informed that a patient has complained to the state board of nursing that a nurse employed with your facility struck him while providing care. What are the legal implications of this information?

   a. What are the ethical implications of this information?

   b. What should be your highest priority action as director of nursing?

9. You are informed that an investigator from the state board of nursing has attempted to contact you as the facility director of nursing to get information about the nurse who has had a complaint brought against her license.

   a. What should be your highest priority action?

   b. If the board of nursing judges there is sufficient cause to pursue the investigation with the nurse, how do you anticipate the process will proceed?

10. You are caring for a woman who is 8 months pregnant and is in a coma after being in a car accident. She is being maintained on a ventilator; the fetus has been shown to be undamaged. What is the ethical conflict in this case and how can it be resolved?

11. You are mentoring a new graduate nurse who expresses concern about giving report to the oncoming shift. He asks you, "Legally, are we allowed to do this? Isn't this a HIPAA violation?" What should be your response? How can you explain to him the major points of the HIPAA law?

NCLEX® Questions

Using the information you obtained from studying this chapter, go online to complete the following NCLEX®-format review questions. Visit http://go.jblearning.com/terryLPN using the access code in the front cover of your book. This interactive resource allows you to answer each question and instantly review your results. Practice until you can answer at least 75% successfully, and then try to improve your score with each successive attempt.

1. An RN is found to be guilty of discriminating against a patient based on that patient's religion. Under the state Nurse Practice Act, the nurse is likely to have discipline brought against his or her license based on
   a. criminal conviction
   b. unprofessional conduct
   c. unethical/unprofessional practice
   d. unsafe practice

2. An RN is found to be guilty of embezzling funds. Under the state Nurse Practice Act, the nurse is likely to have discipline brought against his or her license based on
   a. criminal conviction
   b. unprofessional conduct
   c. unethical/unprofessional practice
   d. unsafe practice

3. An RN is found to be guilty of negligence in his or her nursing practice. Under the state Nurse Practice Act the nurse is likely to have discipline brought against his or her license based on
   a. criminal conviction
   b. unprofessional conduct
   c. unethical/unprofessional practice
   d. unsafe practice

4. An RN is found to be guilty of obtaining a nursing license using a false name. Under the state Nurse Practice Act, the nurse is likely to have discipline brought against his or her license based on
   a. criminal conviction
   b. unprofessional conduct
   c. unethical/unprofessional practice
   d. unsafe practice

5. The RN notes that his patient's chart now includes a document that names another person who can make decisions about the patient's health care if she is unable to do so. The RN recognizes this document as a(n)
   a. living will
   b. durable power of attorney
   c. advanced directive
   d. patient self-determination

6. The RN finds that his patient is asking for information on how to provide some basic instructions on his wishes for health care if he is unable to verbalize what he wants done for himself. The RN recognizes the patient needs to complete a(n)
   a. living will
   b. durable power of attorney
   c. advanced directive
   d. patient self-determination

7. The RN is caring for a patient who arrived at the hospital with a document naming another person to make decisions about her health care if she is unable to do so. The document also provides information describing the circumstances under which the person would want a feeding tube as well as ventilator placement. The RN recognizes that this is a(n)
   a. living will
   b. durable power of attorney
   c. advanced directive
   d. patient self-determination

8. The RN experiences frustration because she reports knowing the right decision to make when caring for dying patients but is prevented from making the right decision by the hospital's policies. This is most likely to be
   a. role conflict
   b. futile care

    c. moral distress

    d. moral courage

9. The unit manager finds the new graduate RN weeping in the break room. The RN tells the unit manager, "I tried so hard to get the doctor to increase Mrs. Jones's pain medication, and now it doesn't help her at all!" The RN is experiencing

    a. role conflict

    b. futile care

    c. moral distress

    d. moral courage

10. The RN experiences stress because the physician has written orders for some expensive supplies to be used in the patient's care although hospital administration has recently issued new policies on financial management. This is known as

    a. role conflict

    b. futile care

    c. moral distress

    d. moral courage

11. The RN takes charge of the evacuation of patients from a hospital that sustained significant storm damage and is able to get everyone to a place of safety. She is demonstrating

    a. role conflict

    b. futile care

    c. moral distress

    d. moral courage

12. The most effective way the RN can demonstrate the ethical principle of veracity is by

    a. not allowing protected health information to be released about the patient

    b. helping the patient understand the nature and extent of his disease process

    c. staying faithful to the nurse–patient relationship

    d. providing the patient with truthful information

Match the description with the correct ethical principle used in nursing.

13. _____ fair and equitable treatment for all patients

14. _____ avoiding misleading patients

15. _____ limiting the amount of information to disclose about oneself

16. _____ information that can be disclosed about a patient without his or her consent

17. _____ being loyal to commitments and accountable for responsibilities

18. _____ avoiding doing harm to the patient

19. _____ the nurse wants to do good for the patient

20. _____ the patient has the right to make his or her own decisions

a. privacy

b. confidentiality

c. veracity

d. fidelity

e. justice

f. nonmaleficence

g. beneficence

h. autonomy

For more information on the topics in this chapter and others, please see Appendix on p. 299 for a list of web links to additional resources.

References

Gallagher, A. (2010). Moral distress and moral courage in everyday nursing practice. *OJIN: Online Journal of Issues in Nursing, 16.* Retrieved from http://www.nursingworld.org/MainMenuCategories/ANAMarketplace /ANAPeriodicals/OJIN/TableofContents/Vol-16-2011/No2-May-2011 /Articles-Previous-Topics/Moral-Distress-and-Courage-in-Everyday-Practice-.html

Huber, D. (2010). *Leadership and nursing care management* (4th ed.). Maryland Heights, MO: Elsevier.

Kelly, P. (2010). *Essentials of nursing leadership and management* (2nd ed.). Clifton Park, NY: Delmar.

Pendry, P. (2007). Recognizing it to retain nurses. *Nursing Economics, 25,* 217–221.

Rumbold, G. (1999). *Ethics in nursing practice* (3rd ed.). New York, NY: Harcourt Brace and Company.

Smith, M. (2009). *Legal basics for professional nursing: Nurse Practice Acts.* Retrieved from http://nursingworld.org/mods/mod995/print.pdf

Wilkinson, J., & Treas, L. (2011). *Fundamentals of nursing* (2nd ed.). Philadelphia, PA: F.A. Davis.

Zerwekh, J., & Garneau, A. (2012). *Nursing today: Transitions and trends* (7th ed.). St. Louis, MO: Elsevier.

For a full suite of assignments and additional learning activities, use the access code located in the front of your book to visit this exclusive website: http://go.jblearning.com/terryLPN. If you do not have an access code, you can obtain one at the site.

www

At the end of this chapter, you will be able to:

1. Discuss the various factors that make up an individual's culture.

2. Describe the various ways a registered nurse can increase his or her cultural competence.

3. Describe beliefs of various cultural or ethnic groups that could affect delivery of nursing care.

4. Discuss the concepts unique to the model of cultural competence in healthcare delivery.

5. Describe the process of conducting a cultural assessment on a patient.

www

KEY TERMS

acculturation
assimilation
biomedical view
cultural awareness
cultural competence
cultural desire

cultural encounters
cultural knowledge
cultural skill
culture
culture shock
Healthy People 2020

holistic view
magico-religious view
socialization
stereotyping
vulnerable populations

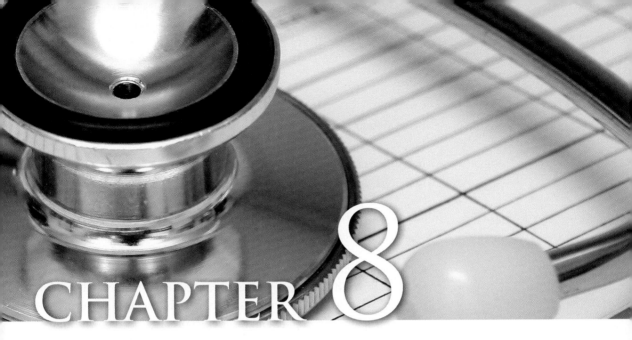

CHAPTER 8

Cultural Aspects of Nursing

Introduction

The registered nurse (RN) transitioning into the healthcare community as a nurse leader must be able to function in not only the local hospital but also in what is increasingly known as the "global society." Americans in particular are multicultural to such an extent that the RN must develop cultural competence to provide adequate nursing care. The nurse who fails to see the importance of being sensitive to a patient's primary language, ethnicity, cultural beliefs, and racial makeup will inevitably provide substandard care because a rapport cannot be built between the nurse and the patient.

Cultural Competence

Cultural competence is the ability to provide care designed specifically for a patient, is inclusive of that patient's cultural norms and values, assists the person in making his or her own decisions regarding health care, and is sensitive to the patient's unique culture (Kelly, 2010). Cultural competence begins with an understanding of culture as a concept. An individual's *culture* is the interwoven pattern of behavior made up of (Kelly, 2010)

< Language
< Thoughts
< Mode of communication
< Actions

< Customs
< Belief system
< Values
< Institutions unique to racial and ethnic makeup
< Religious and social groups

In addition, several things characterize culture as a concept (Wilkinson & Treas, 2011) (**Table 8-1**):

< Culture is learned: The individual learns how to view his or her life and role in it through the other members of the culture. Frequently, the older members of the culture provide instruction to the younger members.
< Culture is taught: The values and beliefs usually are passed down from one generation to the next, with some younger members accepting of the traditional practices and others choosing not to see the value of such teaching.
< Culture is shared by its members: As social interaction occurs with all members of the culture, the concepts that are unique to the culture are passed back and forth.
< Culture is constantly changing: Cultural beliefs and practices change over time; change can occur in response to the culture's environment. This could occur if a culture loses its traditional homeland because of war in the home country.
< Culture is complex: Many cultural concepts occur on an unconscious level and may be difficult for members of the culture to verbalize.
< Culture is diverse: Variety exists among members of a particular cultural group.
< Culture is multilevel: Culture consists of both a material level composed of art, literature, costumes, and artifacts and a nonmaterial level composed of traditions, language, beliefs, and practices.
< Culture is sharing beliefs and practices: For a practice or belief to be considered cultural in nature, it must be shared by the majority of the members of a culture.
< Culture is influential: The culture should be capable of influencing all aspects of members' lives.
< Culture is identifying: Cultural beliefs can provide a sense of belonging for the members even if the culture involved is a subculture; however, if the beliefs of the subculture conflict with the beliefs of the primary culture, the subculture can prove to be a detrimental influence on the members.

TABLE 8-1 Summary of Characteristics of Culture

Characteristic	Description	Meaning for the RN
Multi-faceted	Made up of the individual's language, thoughts, mode of communication, actions, customs, belief system, values, and institutions that are unique to his/her racial and ethnic makeup as well as his/her chosen religious and social groups.	Recognize that the individual's culture is composed of many interconnected parts, each of which is very important.
Learned	The individual learns about how to view his or her life and role in it through the other members of the culture. Frequently the older members of the culture provide instruction to the younger members.	Notice if the older members of the culture are able to successfully pass on traditions and practices to the younger members.
Taught	The values, beliefs, and generations usually are passed down from one generation to the next, with some younger members being accepting of the traditional practices and others choosing not to see the value of such teaching.	Notice if the older members of the culture are able to successfully pass on traditions and practices to the younger members. Determine the beliefs and practices, especially those that are health-related, that are passed down from one generation to the next.
Shared by members	As social interaction occurs with all of the members of the culture, the concepts that are unique to the culture are passed back and forth.	Notice if the older members of the culture are able to successfully pass on traditions and practices to the younger members. Determine the beliefs and practices, especially those that are health-related, that are passed down from one generation to the next. Are there some that seem to be more easily passed down than others?

Characteristic	Description	Meaning for the RN
Constantly changing	Cultural beliefs and practices change over time; change can occur in response to the culture's environment; this could occur if a culture loses its traditional homeland because of war in the home country.	Notice if the cultural beliefs and practices are changing in a positive way or if members are acquiring new but negative beliefs and behavior patterns.
Complex	Many cultural concepts occur on an unconscious level and may be difficult for members of the culture to verbalize.	Spend time with members of the culture who assume leadership roles to grasp the meaning of various aspects of the culture. Many times the older members of the culture will be in leadership positions.
Diverse	Variety exists among members of a particular cultural group.	An example of this would be the gypsy culture, composed of many groups in virtually every nation, speaking many languages and with diverse practices, yet still comprising one overall cultural group. Note the variety that occurs among the members and determine if it is simply physiological diversity or if the cultural group is beginning to be absorbed into the overall larger culture and is disintegrating.
Multilevel	Culture consists of both a material level composed of art, literature, costumes, and artifacts, and a nonmaterial level composed of traditions, language, beliefs, and practices.	An example of this would be a culture that used ceremonial costumes, spoke its own language, generated drawings and stories, and passed on its own traditions to younger generations. Try to get older members of the culture to show you the costumes they were married in, for example. Listen to them speak to each other in their own language.

Characteristic	Description	Meaning for the RN
Sharing beliefs and practices	For a practice or belief to be considered to be cultural in nature, it must be shared by the majority of the members of a culture.	Notice if all of the members have the same belief or practice—if only a few members share the belief, it is not cultural in nature.
Influential	The culture should be capable of influencing all aspects of the members' lives.	The nurse may notice older members of the cultural group being more influenced by the beliefs and practices of the overall group than are younger members. Younger members may be more influenced by their outside peer groups.
Identifying	Cultural beliefs can provide a sense of belonging for the members even if the culture involved is a subculture; however, if the beliefs of the subculture conflict with the beliefs of the primary culture, the subculture can prove to be a detrimental influence on the members.	This sense of belonging can be either positive or negative. It could be positive for a group of immigrants moving from one country to another because it enables them to maintain their identity as a culture. It could be negative when it is applied to an inner city gang that supplies troubled youth with a sense of belonging.

Source: Wilkinson and Treas, 2011; Kelly, 2010.

These factors that form an individual's culture are significant to such an extent that they affect the way in which the person thinks, processes a problem to solve it, and views the world and the way it is structured. Culture is a valuable part of a society because of its ability to communicate past experiences of the group and thus ensure traditions are passed from one generation to the next. This significance can be shown by the *culture shock* that develops when a person emigrates from one culture to another and finds his or her belief system and values are not highly esteemed by the new culture (Kelly, 2010).

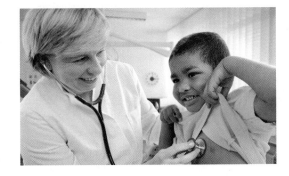

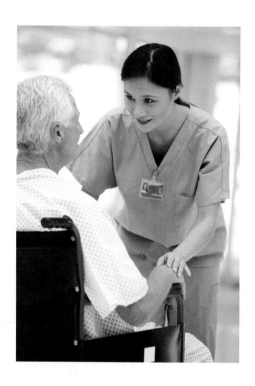

In a society, in addition to the major cultural group to which all individuals belong, we all also belong to multiple smaller subcultures, each with its own belief system and values and expectations for its members. Subcultures you may belong to as a RN may include

< Professional affiliations (RN, American Nurses Association, Sigma Theta Tau International Honor Society for Nursing)
< Age group (middle-aged or older adult)
< Socioeconomic level (middle class)
< Political affiliation (Democratic, Republican, Libertarian)

A person admitted into the modern healthcare system may also experience culture shock, as he or she becomes part of a culture and experiences new words, frightening sights, strange odors, and a never-ending stream of strangers entering his or her personal space. Such culture shock increases greatly when the patient also does not speak English as his or her primary language (Kelly, 2010).

It is important for the RN to increase his or her cultural competence. According to Maddalena (2009), cultural competence can be cultivated to grow and flourish by taking the following actions:

< Examining personal values, behaviors, beliefs, and assumptions, especially as they apply to members of other cultures
< Recognizing evidence of racism in yourself, in coworkers, and in the work environment
< Participating in activities that allow the experiencing of other perspectives and views of the world
< Becoming familiar with primary cultural aspects of the community you serve; learn to recognize what patients from these cultures consider appropriate regarding personal space, physical contact between members of different genders, appropriate social roles for males and females, and expectations for each gender
< Encouraging patients to express how their beliefs and values are different from yours
< Making an effort to learn how various cultures experience health, illness, and treatment

‹ Forging a trusting nurse–patient relationship by exhibiting caring, understanding, and a willingness to listen to other perceptions and viewpoints

Much of this can be accomplished through the use of open-ended communication techniques such as those discussed previously.

Functioning as a Culture

How does a culture actually function in modern society? We must recognize
initially that, as noted in the previous discussion regarding subcultures, almost
no one belongs to only one cultural group. Just as most areas of the United
States are multicultural because they are populated by people from a wide
variety of cultural groups, hospitals and other healthcare environments are
multicultural. They are filled with people from various subcultures: nurses,
physicians, nursing assistants, respiratory therapists, nursing students, and
patients' family members, to name only a few. All these individuals are from
various ethnic groups, races, and religious groups and serve a variety of roles
in society. As these groups gain new members, those individuals must be
socialized into the group by learning how to function as a member of this
cultural group. The nursing student learns how to conduct himself or herself
in the clinical setting, in the classroom, and with other students (Wilkinson
& Treas, 2011).

This process can be more difficult for the person who joins a new cultural
group as an immigrant from another country. The immigrant must adopt the
characteristics of the new culture through *acculturation*, thus assuming aspects
of both cultures. This ensures survival in the new culture associated with the
new country. Some experts have estimated that an immigrant group may require
three generations to become acculturated.

Some immigrant groups take the process one
step further to *assimilation*, in which these individuals choose to learn about and assume the
values, beliefs, and behaviors of the primary
culture of the nation. You could be spoken of as
assimilated into French culture, for example, if
you moved to France, learned to speak French,
began working in the French healthcare system,
became close friends with several French citizens, and learned the French style of cooking
(Wilkinson & Treas, 2011).

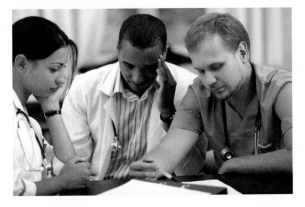

Vulnerable Populations

Vulnerable populations are groups of individuals who are likely to develop health problems and experience poor outcomes in response to nursing interventions and medical treatment as a result of diminished access to medical care, various types of stressors, and engaging in types of high-risk behavior. Such groups can include the following:

- Homeless individuals
- Individuals living below the poverty line
- People experiencing mental illness
- People with various types of physical disabilities and challenges
- Children
- Older adults

Some ethnic and racial minorities are considered to be vulnerable populations because of the known prevalence of various disease processes among them. For example, African Americans are known to have a high rate of hypertension, osteoporosis is prevalent among small-framed White women, and Native Americans and Alaska Natives are known to be vulnerable to develop diabetes (Wilkinson & Treas, 2011).

Healthy People 2020

Healthy People 2020 was developed by the U.S. Department of Health and Human Services (2010) in an attempt to address the gaps in care for vulnerable populations and ultimately to decrease the existing health disparities in America. The project consists of a set of goals and objectives with a 10-year target designed to guide health promotion and disease prevention on a national scale. The basic premise of the initiative is that the combination of goal setting and evidence-based benchmarks can be used to motivate individuals and focus actions designed to improve their health. Healthy People 2020 and its previous versions has been used by the federal government, state governments, and individual communities to measure the progress in resolving health issues in certain vulnerable populations (U.S. Department of Health and Human Services, 2010).

As a public health initiative, Healthy People 2020 identified a mission, as follows (U.S. Department of Health and Human Services, 2010):

- Identify priorities for improving individuals' health throughout the United States

< Increase public awareness of what determines health, disease, and disabling conditions, as well as opportunities to resolve disease processes
< Develop measurable goals and objectives that are useful at the national, state, and community levels
< Involve multiple personnel to act to strengthen policies and improve evidence-based practices
< Identify research, evaluation, and data collection priorities

In addition, the primary goals of Healthy People 2020 are identified as follows:

< Attain lives of greater longevity and higher quality that have no evidence of preventable disease, disability, injury, or premature death
< Achieve equity in health, eliminate evidence of health disparities, and improve the health status of all vulnerable populations
< Create both social and physical environments that promote an overall increased level of health for all individuals involved
< Promote the increased quality of life, healthy development, and health-promoting behaviors across all stages of the life span

The mission and goals of Healthy People 2020 impact the RN nurse leader who is providing care in today's healthcare community. Baldwin (2003) described the demographics of modern America as changing so drastically that it is estimated that by the year 2040 the Hispanic population will increase by 21%, the Asian population by 22%, African Americans by 12%, and Whites by 2%. These figures suggest that modern nurses must be prepared to care for individuals who may reap the benefits of modern medicine in terms of longevity and treatability of conditions but who also may speak English as a second language or not at all (Baldwin, 2003).

Ample documentation in the literature indicates that racial and/or ethnic minority groups are affected by specific disease processes, for example, diabetes mellitus or hypertension, to a greater extent than their White counterparts. This is believed to be the result of the following (Baldwin, 2003):

< Socioeconomic status
< Health behaviors practiced by the various minority groups or the lack thereof
< Access to health care
< Environmental factors such as water supply and crop growth
< Manifestations of discrimination such as job availability

‹ Lack of health insurance

‹ Overdependence on publicly funded facilities

‹ Inadequate transportation

‹ Inadequate numbers of healthcare providers in a specific area

‹ Cost of healthcare services

Leading Causes of Death in Specific Populations

Although the leading causes of death are the same for Whites and for African-Americans (i.e., heart disease, cancer, and stroke), the causes begin to diverge beyond that point. The remaining 10 leading causes of death for Whites are, in order, chronic lower respiratory disease, unintentional injury, influenza and pneumonia, Alzheimer's disease, diabetes, nephritis, and suicide. In comparison, the remaining 10 leading causes of death for African-Americans are, in order, diabetes, unintentional injury, homicide, chronic lower respiratory disease, human immunodeficiency virus, nephritis, and septicemia (Centers for Disease Control and Prevention, 2005).

In addition, former Surgeon General David Satcher estimated that mortality rates in incidence of cardiac disease for African Americans are 40% higher than those for Whites. The death rate for all types of cancer is 30% higher for African Americans than Whites and the rate of prostate cancer in African Americans is more than double that of Whites. The incidence of human immunodeficiency virus is more than seven times that of the incidence for Whites, and the rate of homicide is at least six times greater in African Americans than for Whites (Satcher, 2000).

Other particularly vulnerable populations are immigrants and refugees. These groups are believed to be particularly vulnerable to the development of pandemic influenza. The number of foreign-born individuals living in the United States is projected to increase from 12% in 2005 to 15% in 2015. In 2009 this number amounted to approximately 38 million individuals (Morello and Keating, 2009). When compared with individuals born in the United States, foreign-born individuals are more likely to live in poverty, less likely to have a high school diploma, and less likely to have healthcare coverage.

Undocumented individuals are most likely to experience barriers to access to health care, because these people tend to avoid contact with public officials due to fear of deportation. Foreign-born individuals are known to have a higher prevalence of diabetes, infections, and occupational injuries than American-born residents of the same race and ethnic origin (Truman et al., 2009).

Some foreign-born individuals may receive fewer routine immunizations, use preventive healthcare less frequently, develop some infectious diseases such as tuberculosis at a significantly higher rate, and delay seeking treatment for some infectious disease processes. The health status of immigrants is further challenged by the pressures of adjusting to a new dominant culture; finding employment, particularly when the individual is undocumented; and learning to communicate in a new language (Truman et al., 2009).

The Hispanic population constitutes an additional vulnerable population with a wide range of health disparities. In 2007 only 41.7% of Hispanics under the age of 65 had private health insurance, whereas 76.2% of Whites were able to obtain it. Hispanic or Latina women were found to be more than twice as likely as White women to have either late prenatal care or no prenatal care at all. Also in 2007, whereas Whites had a rate of 51.3% for influenza vaccination for adults over the age of 18, Hispanic or Latino adults had a rate of 35.5%. Furthermore, when the rate of immunization against pneumococcal vaccination coverage was considered, the rate for Hispanics was half that of Whites. The death rate from diabetes among Hispanics was found to be almost 1.5 times higher than for Whites. Among Hispanics, the highest death rate was among Puerto Ricans, followed by Mexican Americans and Cuban Americans. When considering all men aged 20 to 74, Mexican Americans were found to have a higher prevalence of being overweight as well as obese than either White or African American men (Centers for Disease Control and Prevention, 2010).

The implications for recognizing that such health problems exist in vulnerable populations are great. There are several strategies to resolve such disparities (Baldwin, 2003):

< Develop prevention programs in the community that involve working with and being connected to a facility; this ensures patients can readily have lab work drawn or nutritional counseling implemented.
< Use the strategies for prevention that have already been discussed; regardless of your role in the overall healthcare continuum, the primary prevention strategies can be practiced by everyone.
< Promote wellness and a healthy lifestyle; be mindful that the healthcare professional must have completed a full assessment of the cultural beliefs and practices of the vulnerable population in question before implementing wellness prevention, as some Western strategies might prove offensive to other cultures.
< Be mindful of the personal choices of individuals and the existing social environment, particularly interactions with family, acquaintances, and

the community; it may prove helpful to involve entire families or even communities in educational sessions.

< Make the effort to provide patients with complete information without seeming to rush the interaction; members of vulnerable populations frequently note that healthcare professionals seem rushed in their interaction with patients, and members of other cultures often find this offensive.

Model of Cultural Competence in Healthcare Delivery

The process of developing cultural competence as part of recognizing the health problems of certain cultural groups can be expedited by the use of open-ended communication skills. It can also be assisted by the use of a nursing model developed by Josepha Campinha-Bacote (2002). This model proposes basic assumptions related to the process of developing cultural competence as a nurse:

< Cultural competence is a gradual process.
< Five concepts are central to the development of cultural competence:
  < Cultural awareness
  < Cultural knowledge
  < Cultural skill
  < Cultural encounters
  < Cultural desire
< More variation occurs within ethnic groups than across ethnic groups.
< A direct relationship exists between the level of competence of a healthcare provider and his or her ability to provide culturally competent health care.
< Cultural competence is essential to the provision of appropriate and sensitive healthcare services to clients who are culturally and/or ethnically diverse.

The major concepts central to Campinha-Bacote's model require discussion to streamline the process of developing cultural competence. *Cultural awareness* is considered to be an examination and exploration of the nurse's cultural and professional background that results in recognizing the nurse's biases, prejudices, and assumptions about people who are different. A nurse who is unaware of his or her own cultural or professional values could potentially impose his or her values on a patient of another culture (Campinha-Bacote, 2002).

In conjunction with the development of cultural awareness is the development of *cultural knowledge*. This is acquired through the process of obtaining research-based information about different cultures and ethnic groups. This information should focus most intensely on obtaining information pertaining to health-related beliefs and cultural values, disease incidence and prevalence in specific cultural or ethnic groups, and treatments that have been used most effectively. When the nurse takes the time to gain information about the patient's health-related beliefs and values, the nurse also gains information about the patient's worldview and conducts a cultural assessment. This will explain how the patient thinks about his or her illness (Campinha-Bacote, 2002).

Cultural skill is the ability to not only accurately perform a cultural assessment but to also collect relevant cultural data about the patient's current problem. The nurse should recognize how the differences in a patient's physical characteristics and biological differences influence the nurse's ability to accurately perform an assessment of the patient (Campinha-Bacote, 2002).

The *cultural encounter* is used by the nurse to interact with a patient from a different cultural background. Interacting and communicating with patients from other cultures will cause the RN to change his or her current beliefs about a cultural group and help the nurse avoid stereotyping the patient. *Stereotyping* occurs when the nurse develops a distorted view of a particular group of people (Huber, 2010). Part of the cultural encounter is an assessment of the language needs of the patient. Consider using a trained interpreter if one is available in the facility because use of friends or family members may prove to be problematic if they are unfamiliar with medical terms (Campinha-Bacote, 2002).

Finally, *cultural desire* is the nurse's motivation to become culturally aware, knowledgeable, and skillful and also encompasses the concept of caring. This motivation is demonstrated by the nurse's genuine need to be accepting of the differences of patients because of the opportunity to learn from them (Campinha-Bacote, 2002).

As the nurse develops cultural knowledge, a great deal of information can be acquired. The nurse should carefully note cultural and spiritual beliefs that are unique to a culture and that could affect the delivery of nursing care. Sensitivity to these beliefs contributes to the development of cultural desire. These beliefs are arranged according to ethnic or cultural group and are shown in **Table 8-2**.

TABLE 8-2 Cultural and Spiritual Beliefs That Could Affect Delivery of Nursing Care

Cultural/Ethnic Group	Beliefs	Nursing Actions
African-American	Extended family will influence the patient. Older family members are honored and respected. The oldest male may serve as the decision-maker for the family.	Involve extended family in teaching sessions. Show respect to older family members. Involve oldest male in the family in making decisions about the family.
Chinese	Will tend to avoid discussing symptoms of mental illness. Will favor use of herbalists and spiritual healers along with physicians.	Avoid appearing to view herbalists and spiritual healers negatively in case the patient has already incorporated them into his or her healthcare regimen.
Japanese	Will avoid discussing issues related to disability, mental illness, pain, or addiction. Health concerns may be brought before the family group when decisions need to be made. Will use physicians, healers, as well as herbalists to treat illness and are unlikely to question care delivered by a physician. Believe that illness can be the result of inadequate diet or lack of sleep.	Involve extended family in teaching sessions. Avoid appearing to view herbalists and spiritual healers negatively in case the patient has already incorporated them into his or her healthcare regimen. Encourage the patient to verbalize to the nurse questions and concerns about the physician's treatment regimen so that these can then be brought to the physician's attention.
Hindu and Muslim	Tend to blend modern healthcare beliefs with traditional practices. May avoid acknowledging family members' evidence of mental illness or intellectual disability because of fear that it will affect chances of other members of the family being able to marry.	Do not attempt to force family members' acknowledgement of mental illness or intellectual disability; make them aware of various resources in the community that would provide assistance for them and the individual.

Cultural/Ethnic Group	Beliefs	Nursing Actions
Vietnamese	May try various home remedies before seeking out Western medicine. Must establish a trusting relationship with a health-care provider before assistance will be accepted. Society is patriarchal in nature and thus the primary male in the household may make decisions for the family.	Several visits may be required to establish the trusting relationship before nursing interventions will be accepted. The nurse may initially have to establish the trust of the primary male in the household. Ask respectfully about the various home remedies that the patient tried before seeking out Western health care.
Hispanic/Latino	Older family members tend to be consulted when decisions must be made involving health and illness. Society is patriarchal in nature and thus the primary male in the household may make decisions for the family. Illness may be seen as divine intervention in response to an exhibition of sinful behavior. Home remedies and folk healers may have been used prior to seeking out Western medicine. May believe that disease is the result of a imbalance in the person's "hot" and "cold" in his body.	Ask respectfully about the various home remedies that the patient tried before seeking out Western health care. Involve extended family in teaching sessions. Show respect to older family members. Involve oldest male in the family in making decisions about the family. May need to work with the local religious entity if patient firmly believes that his illness is divinely caused.
Asian/Pacific Islander	There usually will be a primary family member who is consulted when significant health-related decisions must be made. Illness is seen as being either divine retribution or the result of supernatural forces. Illness is viewed as being preventable through a combination of nutrition, herbs, rest, cleanliness, laxative use, and the use of both copper and silver bracelets.	Identify the family member who must be consulted regarding health-related decisions and show respect during interactions with this individual. Avoid appearing skeptical when discussing patient's use of copper or silver bracelets to prevent illness. May need to work with the local religious entity if patient firmly believes that his illness is divinely caused.

Cultural/Ethnic Group	Beliefs	Nursing Actions
American Indian	Patient will tend to think only in the present, and will have difficulty with instructions regarding something to do in the future. Will tend to believe that the person is in a healthy state when he is in harmony with nature, and thus illness occurs when there is a balance between the patient and nature or the supernatural. There may be a mistrust of healthcare providers, and thus a medicine man or medicine woman may be consulted initially.	Do not attempt to give patient an extensive schedule of health-related practices that extends beyond the present time. Avoid appearing skeptical when discussing patient's use of a medicine man or his concern regarding a "balanced" state.

Source: Zerwekh & Garneau, 2012.

Once the nurse has made the effort to understand the cultural beliefs of the patient, the process of communication can begin. Multiple cultural-related factors will affect communication with the patient (D'Amico and Barbarito, 2007) (**Table 8-3**):

< Dominant spoken and written language: According to census data released in 2007, 20% of the American population spoke a language other than English (Ohlemacher, 2007). Furthermore, even among English-speaking individuals, there are differences in word use and pronunciation, and various tones of voice can be considered more significant than others.

< Methods of nonverbal communication: These include gestures, facial expressions, and various types of mannerisms. Emotions can be communicated nonverbally through the use of silence, touch, eye contact or failure to make eye contact, moving away from others during the process of communication, and posture of the speaker or listener. It is important to recognize which cultures value silence as demonstrating respect for another individual and which ones use silence to indicate interest in the speaker's words. Also, some cultures do not allow casual

touch and also have strict requirements regarding personal space. Some have specific rules regarding what type of touch is considered to be appropriate for members of the opposite gender.

‹ Time orientation: A culture may have unique views of the past, present, and future. Whereas European Americans view time in terms of

TABLE 8-3 Cultural-Related Factors That Could Affect Communication with the Patient

Factor	Description	Nursing Actions
Dominant spoken and written language	At least 14% of the American population speak Spanish, French, Creole, German, Italian, or some form of Asian or Pacific Island language. Furthermore, even among English-speaking individuals, there are differences in word use and pronunciation, and various tones of voice can be considered more significant than others.	Be sensitive to the patient's cultural beliefs regarding appropriate word use and voice tone. Support patient's need to communicate in his or her dominant language; try to use trained interpreter when there is the need to explain complicated medical procedures to the patient.
Methods of nonverbal communication	These include gestures, facial expressions, and various types of mannerisms. Emotions can be communicated nonverbally through use of silence, touch, eye contact or failure to make eye contact, moving away from others during communication, as well as posture of the speaker as well as the listener. Recognize which cultures value silence as demonstrating respect for another individual and which ones use silence to indicate interest in the speaker's words. Also, some cultures do not allow casual touch and have strict requirements regarding personal space. Some have specific rules regarding type of touch considered appropriate for members of the opposite gender.	Be sensitive to the patient's cultural beliefs regarding use of silence, touch that is considered appropriate between genders, and the use of eye contact. Identify methods of nonverbal communication that are considered to be appropriate and inappropriate.

Factor	Description	Nursing Actions
Time orientation	A culture may have unique views of the past, present, and future. Whereas European Americans view time in terms of punctuality and scheduling, other cultures are not as future oriented. For example, some American Indians consider time primarily in terms of the past. Time is important to them because of the traditional practices that have been passed down through generations from their ancestors. In comparison, some Hispanic cultures do not view time as being as significant.	Determine the culture's view of time and orientation as to past, present, or future. The nurse may need to use shorter-range planning with a client who has difficulty with long-range planning. Plan to review important points at frequent intervals for emphasis. Determine if tools such as large-view calendars are more effective than those such as medication planners that require more manual dexterity.
Family roles and relationships	The specified roles and relationships in the patient's family relate to how decision-making is valued and implemented, the culture's view of age as well as specific views of each gender. Some cultures are more likely to follow a patriarchal or matriarchal pattern of decision-making.	Determine if the patient's family has a patriarchal or matriarchal view of decision-making. Demonstrate respect for the older members of the patient's family. Identify if there are members of the family who are especially significant regarding decision-making.
Nutritional intake	The patient's daily diet may be culturally determined. Specific foods may be eaten at specific times or as part of cultural ritualistic practices. The RN should familiarize himself or herself with as many of these as possible since they can significantly affect the patient's treatment and recovery process. They can include: a. Americans typically have coffee in the morning with breakfast b. Muslims will fast from dawn to sunset during the month of Ramadan as part of their religious practice	Identify foods considered to be appropriate for the patient based on cultural beliefs and requirements. Determine if facility can appropriately meet the dietary needs of the patient from a cultural and/or religious standpoint. Determine if patient believes that certain foods can contribute to his recovery, such as in the balance between hot and cold foods.

Factor	Description	Nursing Actions
	c. Roman Catholics will observe Lent by eating one full meal and two small meals on Ash Wednesday and Good Friday, and will avoid eating meat on Ash Wednesday and Fridays until Easter as part of their religious practice d. Muslims avoid eating pork e. Jews may practice kosher dietary laws, and f. Mexican, Iranian, Chinese, and Vietnamese cultures all view achieving the balance between hot and cold foods as both a method of preventing illness and a method of treating illness.	
Types of religious beliefs/health practices	Health beliefs will typically fall into one of three types: *magico-religious*, *biomedical*, or *holistic*. The magico-religious view holds that health and illness are the result of supernatural intervention. The biomedical view proposes that illness is caused by germs, viruses, or some type of breakdown in the basic functioning of the body. The holistic type of health beliefs propose that illness results from man's life failing to be in harmony with nature.	Identify the source of the client's cultural health beliefs. Avoid appearing skeptical if the source of client's health beliefs is significantly different from that of the nurse.

Source: D'Amico & Barbarito, 2007.

punctuality and scheduling, other cultures are not as future oriented. For example, some Native Americans consider time primarily in terms of the past. Time is important to them because of the traditional practices that have been passed down through generations from their ancestors. In comparison, some Hispanic cultures do not view time as significant.

Family roles and relationships: The specified roles and relationships in the patient's family relate to how decision-making is valued and

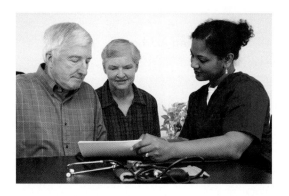

implemented, the culture's view of age, and specific views of each gender. Some cultures are more likely to follow a patriarchal pattern of decision-making, whereas others tend to consult the matriarchal member of the family for assistance with decision-making.

< Nutritional intake: The patient's daily diet may be culturally determined. Specific foods may be eaten at specific times or as part of cultural ritualistic practices. The RN should familiarize himself or herself with as many of these as possible because they can significantly affect the patient's treatment and recovery process:

< Americans typically have coffee in the morning with breakfast.

< Muslims fast from dawn to sunset during the month of Ramadan as part of their religious practice.

< Roman Catholics observe Lent by eating one full meal and two small meals on Ash Wednesday and Good Friday and avoid eating meat on Ash Wednesday and Fridays until Easter as part of their religious practice.

< Muslims avoid eating pork.

< Jews may practice kosher dietary laws.

< Mexican, Iranian, Chinese, and Vietnamese cultures all view achieving the balance between hot and cold foods as both a method of preventing illness and a method of treating illness.

< Types of health beliefs and health practices: Health beliefs typically fall into one of three types: *magico-religious*, *biomedical*, or *holistic*. The magico-religious view holds that health and illness are the result of supernatural intervention. The biomedical view proposes that illness is caused by germs, viruses, or some type of breakdown in the basic functioning of the body. The holistic view proposes that illness results from a person's life failing to be in harmony with nature.

Summary of Key Points in Chapter

The chapter discussed various aspects of assessing and caring for a patient of another culture. The factors that make up the concept of culture were reviewed, as well as the need for cultural competence from the RN. In addition, ways for the nurse to increase cultural competence in providing care to the patient were discussed.

The process of conducting a cultural assessment was described as part of verifying the existence of various health inequities in vulnerable populations of patients. The concepts unique to the model of cultural competence in healthcare delivery as a method of increasing the nurse's degree of cultural competence were discussed.

Finally, the health disparities present in various vulnerable populations of patients were described, specifically the cultural or ethnic minorities of

< African-American population
< Hispanic population
< Immigrant/refugee population

Conclusion

Regardless of the role implemented in the modern healthcare facility or simply in the current healthcare continuum, today's RN has surely noted that he or she is serving the current healthcare customer in a global society. The RN in a busy metropolitan hospital is just as likely to be working with a patient from Nigeria as one from the local community. Because of the existence of the modern global society, RNs must recognize the need to develop a high level of cultural competence and the capability to perform a thorough cultural assessment on a patient. Without such knowledge, the professional will lack the ability to quickly detect health problems in a patient's societal group and may inadvertently allow a patient to do without much-needed health care.

A huge part of working with patients from other cultures is establishing the nurse–patient relationship, which is forged on the trust that the patient has in the abilities of the nurse. This trust will develop as the nurse cares for the patient consistently and accurately. Much of this trust will grow as the patient observes the nurse calculating and administering medication dosages accurately. Procedures for dosage and solution calculation are discussed in the next chapter.

Critical Thinking Questions

1. List as many things as you can that make up your own individual culture.

2. Describe an incident when you experienced culture shock and your reaction to it.

3. Try to list all the subcultures to which you belong.

4. Look at the list of the subcultures you developed in question 3. How has being part of each subculture affected your beliefs and values?

5. Consider your current or former work environment.
   a. Can you recall a time when you observed a patient experiencing culture shock?
   b. What was the outcome of this experience?

6. Compare and contrast cultural awareness, cultural knowledge, cultural skill, cultural encounters, and cultural desire.

7. Consider the most effective way to resolve the following situations: Your patient is complaining he is unable to obtain the type of dietary intake that meets the requirements of his culture while he is hospitalized. What can you do to resolve this so that
   a. the patient receives the food that is culturally correct?
   b. the dietary staff understands what is culturally appropriate for the patient's dietary intake?
   c. the patient's family is involved in planning the patient's dietary intake?
   d. the hospital does not go to an excessive amount of expense because of the patient's cultural dietary requirements?

8. The hospital where you work cannot afford either to hire a trained interpreter to work with its large population of Korean-speaking patients or to send an employee for the required training needed. You are the nurse manager of the medical floor where many of the Korean-speaking patients usually are admitted.
   a. What can you do to communicate with these patients more effectively?
   b. You find that the number of Korean-speaking patients admitted to your floor is increasing. What resources can you find in your community that would help you communicate more effectively with these patients and also help you understand the culture?

9. The one nurse in the facility who speaks fluent Spanish where you are employed is out on medical leave. A tour bus with 20 Spanish-speaking tourists has been involved in an accident and 12 passengers have been brought to your hospital's emergency department. What can you do to most effectively communicate with patients in this situation?

10. How can you most effectively perform triage in the emergency department with this large group of Spanish-speaking patients?

Scenarios

1. You are caring for a 21-year-old Hispanic woman admitted to your medical floor after gashing her leg badly in a car accident. At her bedside is her 30-year-old husband who is assuming the role of interpreter. The patient understands most English that is spoken to her but can speak very little. She has been able to communicate with you so far that she is in a great deal of pain and is concerned about her three children, ages 4, 3, and 6 months.

   a. Describe what you would do to develop cultural awareness as part of the process of becoming culturally competent in caring for this patient.

   b. Describe what you would do to develop cultural knowledge as part of the process of becoming culturally competent in caring for this patient.

   c. Describe what you would do to develop cultural skills as part of the process of becoming culturally competent in caring for this patient.

   d. Describe what you would do to experience cultural encounters as part of the process of becoming culturally competent in caring for this patient.

   e. Describe what you would do to develop cultural desire as part of the process of becoming culturally competent in caring for this patient.

2. You are caring for a patient who is a 48-year-old Pacific Islander. He is a newly diagnosed diabetic, is 25 pounds overweight, and is married and has 2 children, ages 14 and 10. He seems very depressed even though the physician believes the diabetes is easily treatable with diet and exercise. What can the nurse do to communicate effectively with the patient and his family?

3. You are working with a 58-year-old female Chinese patient who is experiencing episodes of severe abdominal pain. She arrives at the health clinical accompanied by her husband, her married daughter, and her grandchildren. The entire family is very concerned and anxious about her situation. What can you do to communicate effectively with this patient and her family?

4. A 72-year-old Japanese patient is brought to the emergency department after sustaining a massive heart attack. In talking with the family you discover the patient had been experiencing pain for at least the past 2 weeks but had been self-medicating with acupuncture treatments. What should you do to communicate effectively with this patient and his family?

5. A 21-year-old Hindu woman is brought into the emergency department after attempting suicide. She is accompanied by her mother who acknowledges that the girl has been experiencing symptoms of depression since being notified that a traditional marriage was being arranged for her by her father. What should you do to communicate effectively with this patient and her family?

6. You are caring for a 48-year-old Hispanic woman who is refusing to receive treatment for ovarian cancer. She tells you the cancer is God's judgment on her for separating from her husband 2 years ago. What should you do to communicate effectively with this patient and her family?

7. You need to teach your Native American patient how to perform a dressing change on his leg wound. The dressing procedure will need to change over the next 2 weeks as the wound progressively heals. What is the best way to teach this patient how to perform the dressing change and care for his leg wound?

8. You are working with a Japanese patient who is recovering from a severe burn. He is refusing opioid pain medication even when he clearly is in severe discomfort. What should you do to communicate effectively with this patient and his family?

9. You are working with an Orthodox Jewish client who observes kosher dietary practices. Which factors do you believe will affect your communication with this patient?

10. You are working with a Muslim patient. Which factors do you believe will affect your communication with this patient?

11. You are working with a Native American patient. Which factors do you believe will affect your communication with this patient?

12. You are working with a Chinese patient who is also blind. Which factors do you believe will affect your communication with this patient?

NCLEX® Questions

Using the information you obtained from studying this chapter, go online to complete the following NCLEX®-format review questions. Visit http://go.jblearning.com/terryLPN using the access code in the front cover of your book. This interactive resource allows you to answer each question and instantly review your results. Practice until you can answer at least 75% successfully, and then try to improve your score with each successive attempt.

Match the cultural/spiritual belief with the appropriate cultural/ethnic group. More than one group can be selected if appropriate.

1. _____ oldest male may serve as the decision-maker for the family
2. _____ patient will tend to think only in the present
3. _____ disease is the result of an imbalance in the patient's "hot" and "cold"
4. _____ trusting relationship must be established with healthcare provider before assistance is accepted
5. _____ may try various home remedies before seeking out Western medicine
6. _____ illness is divine intervention in response to sinful behavior
7. _____ older family members are consulted about decisions involved health and illness
8. _____ may avoid acknowledging family members' evidence of mental illness or intellectual disability for fear it will affect chances of other family members' ability to marry
9. _____ patient will have difficulty with instructions regarding something to do in the future
10. _____ illness can be the result of inadequate diet or lack of sleep
11. _____ illness can be prevented through the use of nutrition, herbs, rest, cleanliness, and laxative use
12. _____ the patient is in a healthy state when he or she is in harmony with nature
13. _____ illness can be prevented through the use of both copper and silver bracelets
14. _____ illness occurs when there is a balance between the patient and nature or the supernatural
15. _____ time is not significant
16. _____ hot and cold foods can be used as a method of preventing and treating illness
17. _____ medicine man or woman may be consulted before healthcare providers
18. _____ time is viewed as being primarily in the past
19. _____ a primary family member may be consulted when significant health-related decisions must be made
20. _____ herbalists and spiritual healers are used along with physicians

a. African American
b. Chinese
c. Japanese
d. Hindu/Muslim
e. Vietnamese

    f. Hispanic/Latino

    g. Asian/Pacific Islander

    h. Native American

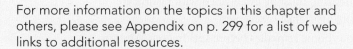

For more information on the topics in this chapter and others, please see Appendix on p. 299 for a list of web links to additional resources.

References

Baldwin, D. (2003). Disparities in health and health care: Focusing efforts to eliminate unequal burdens. *Online Journal of Issues in Nursing, 8.* Retrieved from www.nursingworld.org/MainMenuCategories/ANAMarketplace /ANAPeriodicals/OJIN/TableofContents/Volume82003/No1Jan2003 /DisparitiesinHealthandHealthCare.aspx

Campinha-Bacote, J. (2002). The process of cultural competence in the delivery of healthcare services: A model of care. *Journal of Transcultural Nursing, 13,* 181–184.

Centers for Disease Control and Prevention. (2005). Health disparities experienced by Black or African Americans—United States. Retrieved from http:// www.cdc.gov/mmwr/preview/mmwrhtml/mm5401a1.htm#tab

Centers for Disease Control and Prevention. (2010). Highlights for minority health and health disparities. Retrieved from http://www.cdc.gov/omhd /Highlights/2010/HSeptOct10.html#DISPARITIES

D'Amico, D., & Barbarito, C. (2007). *Health and physical assessment in nursing.* Upper Saddle River, NJ: Pearson.

Huber, D. (2010). *Leadership and nursing care management* (4th ed.). Maryland Heights, MO: Elsevier.

Kelly, P. (2010). *Essentials of nursing leadership and management* (2nd ed.). Clifton Park, NY: Delmar.

Maddalena, V. (2009). Cultural competence and holistic practice: Implications for education, practice, and research. *Holistic Nursing Practice, 23,* 153–157.

Morello, C. and Keating, D. (September 22, 2009). Number of foreign-born U.S. residents drops. *The Washington Post.* Retrieved from http://www.washington post.com/wpdyn/content/article/2009/09/21/AR2009092103251.html

Ohlemacher, S. (2007, September 12). 20 percent of people living in U.S. speak language other than English at home. *The Post and Courier.* Retrieved from http://www.postandcourier.com/news/2007/sep/12/language15626/

Satcher, D. (2000, May 11). *U.S. Public Health Service, Department of Health and Human Services before the House Commerce Committee*: Subcommittee on Health and Environment. Washington, DC: U.S. Public Health Service, Department of Health and Human Services.

Truman, B., Tinker, T., Vaughan, E., Kapella, B., Brenden, M., Woznica, C., … Lichveld, M. (2009). Pandemic influenza preparedness and response among immigrants and refugees. *American Journal of Public Health, 99,* S278–S286.

U.S. Department of Health and Human Services. (2010, November). *Healthy People 2020.* Retrieved from http://www.healthypeople.gov/2020/Topics Objectives2020/pdfs/HP2020_brochure.pdf

Wilkinson, J., & Treas, L. (2011). *Fundamentals of nursing* (2nd ed.). Philadelphia, PA: F.A. Davis.

For a full suite of assignments and additional learning activities, use the access code located in the front of your book to visit this exclusive website: http://go.jblearning.com/terryLPN. If you do not have an access code, you can obtain one at the site.

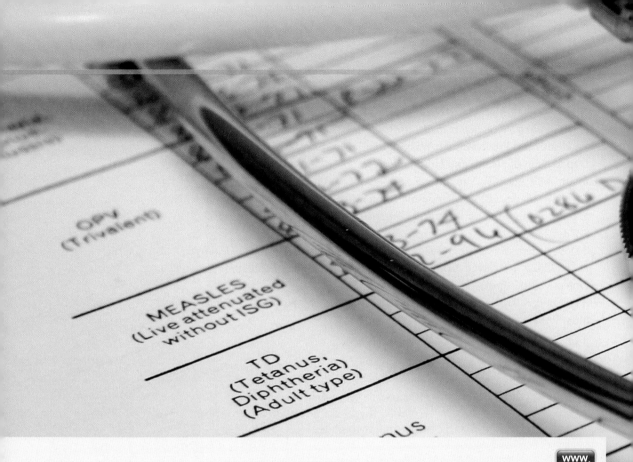
(Live attenuated
without ISG)

OPV
(Trivalent)

MEASLES
(Live attenuated
without ISG)

TD
(Tetanus,
Diphtheria)
(Adult type)

CHAPTER OBJECTIVES

At the end of this chapter, you will be able to:

1. Identify common conversion factors used in calculating dosages and solutions.

2. Become familiar with the ratio and proportion method of calculating dosages and solutions.

3. Become familiar with the "desired over available" method of calculating dosages and solutions.

4. Become familiar with the dimensional analysis method of calculating dosages and solutions.

5. Become familiar with the various formulas used in calculating flow rates and infusion times of intravenous dosages and solutions.

KEY TERMS

Clark's rule
drop factor
flow rate

Fried's rule
proportion

ratio
Young's rule

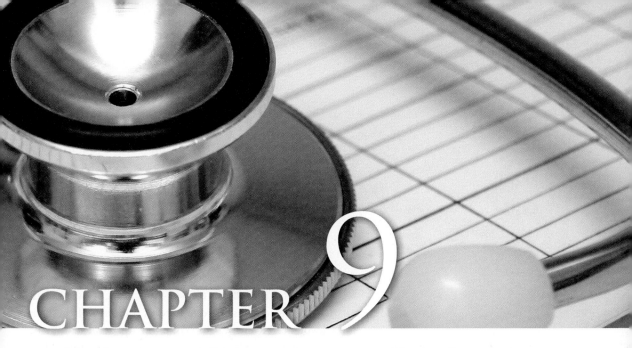

CHAPTER 9

Calculation of Dosages and Solutions

Introduction

In today's modern healthcare environment the registered nurse holds a vast amount of responsibility and literally can make the difference in whether a patient lives or dies. The nurse's ability to calculate dosages and solutions of medications can vastly improve the patient's odds of leaving the hospital setting with his or her quality of life not only maintained but even enhanced. Here, various methods of calculating dosages and solutions are reviewed along with important conversion factors, formulas, and other information forming a knowledge base for this topic.

Conversion Factors

When first confronted with a dosage problem that requires calculation, initially read the problem or review the information on the drug label closely. Can you clearly locate the following?

- The amount of the drug found in each tablet, capsule, or milliliter of medication, for example, "500 mg of medication per 1 tablet." This is what you have on hand.
- Additional information needed, such as the solvent needed to dissolve a powdered medication. The manufacturer will list the solution recommended to dissolve the medication, for example, "add 10 ml 0.9% normal saline to yield 500 mg of the drug per 1 ml of solution."

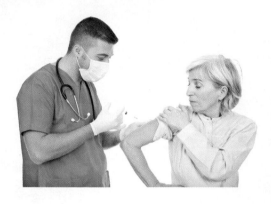

Also review the physician's order for the dosage problem, if available, or the medication administration record. If you cannot determine from the physician's order what the patient is to be given, the physician should be contacted for additional clarification. If the directions for preparing the medication are confusing, contact the facility pharmacy for assistance.

Once you have clarified what has been ordered for the patient along with what you have on hand, determine if the unit of measurement of the drug ordered for the patient is the same as the one used in the form of the drug available to you. If not, you need to convert to a common unit of measurement. This means, for example, that if the physician orders an amount of medication in milligrams but the pharmacy has the medication available in a form that is measured in grains, the nurse will need to convert the ordered amount to grains, the form of the drug the pharmacy has on hand. The following is a list of frequently used, common conversion factors (Curren, 2008):

1 cup (c) = 8 ounces (oz)

1 dram (dr) = 60 grains (gr)

1 dram (fl dr) = 60 minims

1 gallon (gal) = 4 quarts (qt)

1 glass = 8 ounces (oz)

1 grain (gr) = 60 milligrams (mg)

1 gram (g) = 15 grains (gr)

1 inch (in) = 2.54 centimeters (cm)

1 kilogram (kg) = 2.2 pounds (lb)

1 ounce (oz) = 2 tablespoons (tbsp)

1 ounce (oz) = 8 drams (dr)

1 pint (pt) = 16 ounces (oz)

1 pound (lb) = 16 ounces (oz)

1 tablespoon (tbsp) = 3 teaspoons (tsp)

1 cubic centimeter (cc) = 1 milliliter (ml)

Ratio and Proportion Method

The ratio and proportion method can be an easy way to begin working problems based on conversion factors. A *ratio* is basically a relationship of two things (in this case, numbers) that exists in terms of size, amount, or quantity. A *proportion* is an equation with a ratio on each side of the equal sign (Burke, 2005). To use these concepts in calculating a problem, consider the following example:

$$30 \text{ mg} = \underline{\hspace{1cm}} \text{ gr}$$

To begin working the problem, first review the problem to determine what you are being asked. You have two different units of measurement, milligram and grains. You can convert to a common unit of measurement by using the ratio and proportion method of calculation.

Second, set up your ratio by writing down the only thing you know for certain. Because you are working with both milligrams and grains, what you know for certain is that 1 grain = 60 mg is the conversion factor. Therefore, write the first half of the problem as

$$1 \text{ gr} : 60 \text{ mg}$$

Once you've written what you know, then write the other half of the proportion, which is what you *don't* know for certain. What you don't know for certain is what you are searching for, which is how many grains of medication are found in 30 mg. You can format that section of the proportion as

$$x \text{ gr} : 30 \text{ mg}$$

The proportion to be solved will ultimately look like this:

$$1 \text{ gr} : 60 \text{ mg} :: x \text{ gr} : 30 \text{ mg}$$

This would be read as

"1 grain is to 60 milligrams as x grains is to 30 milligrams"

You'll cross-multiply to solve the equation so the problem will be calculated as

$$1 \text{ gr} : 60 \text{ mg} :: x \text{ gr} : 30 \text{ mg}$$

This means the problem is now calculated as $60x = 30$. This introduces a concept unique to the ratio and proportion method of solving dosage and solution problems: the "means" and the "extremes." The "means" are the two inner numbers of the proportion, in this case, 60 and x. The "extremes" are the two outer numbers of the proportion, in this case, 1 and 30. The means must always be multiplied together and the extremes must be multiplied together. If you ever inadvertently multiply the means and the extreme in such a way that the means or the extremes are not multiplied together, stop calculating and go back to your proportion to clarify how the numbers should have been multiplied.

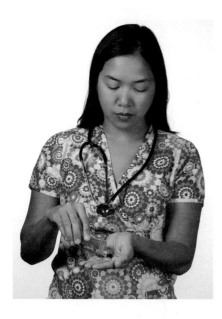

Remember that the side of the calculation where "*x*" is found is important, because this is the unknown factor for which you are searching. You're always solving for *x*. To do this, *x* must stand alone. Therefore, you must divide by the number on the same side as *x* in order for *x* to stand by itself. In the case of the example, you'll be dividing by 60, like this: 60*x*/60 = 30. When you reach this point of a calculation, always remember that whatever you do to one side of the calculation must be also performed on the other side of the calculation, like this: 60*x*/60 = 30/60. On the left side of this proportion, 60/60 equals 1, thus making the left side simply become *x*. On the right side of the proportion, 30/60 becomes ½. Therefore, *x* = ½. To solve the problem, we need to go back to the original question that was asked: 30 mg = _____ gr. According to our calculation, 30 mg = ½ gr. We can verify this answer by going back to our conversions and finding that 1 grain = 60 milligrams; therefore, ½ grain = 30 milligrams.

Calculate the following conversion problems using the ratio and proportion method.

1. ½ fluid ounce = ___ml
2. 1.4 g = _____mcg
3. 2 tbsp = _____ml
4. 3 liters = _____ml
5. 3 oz = _____tbsp
6. 1.5 tsp = _____ml
7. gr v = _____mg
8. 10 kg = _____lb
9. 0.25 g = _____mg
10. gr 1/200 = _____mg

Answers:

1. 15 ml
2. 1,400,000 mcg
3. 30 ml
4. 3,000 ml
5. 6 tbsp
6. 7.5 ml
7. 300 mg
8. 22 lbs

9. 250 mg

10. 0.3 mg

From Math for Meds, (Curren, 2008)

Desired Over Available Method

Before using this method of calculation, it is imperative that you perform whatever conversion is necessary to ensure the same units of measurement are used. If you realize this step has not been performed, stop the calculation.

In this formula three concepts are used:

D = desired dose or ordered dose

H = dose available or "on hand"

V = vehicle or form of the drug available, whether tablet or liquid

The basic formula is

$$\frac{D \times V}{H}$$

You could use this formula to work dosage and solution problems in the following manner. Let's assume the physician has written an order for drug A 50 mg three times daily. You have available to you 125 mg of the medication per 5 ml of liquid medication. How much medication should you prepare to administer 50 mg? The desired dose is 50 mg, the dosage on hand is 125 mg, and the vehicle is 5 ml, so the calculation is written as (Diehl, 2010)

$$\frac{50 \times 5}{125} = \frac{250}{125} = 2 \text{ ml}$$

Calculate the following problems using the desired over available method.

1. The doctor has ordered drug A 15 mg. You have 10 mg drug A tablets on hand. How many tablets do you give?

2. The doctor has ordered drug B 300 mg. You have drug B 900 mg in 6 ml. How many ml do you administer?

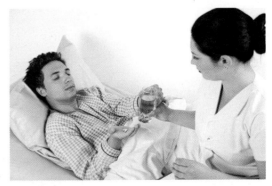

College of the Ouachitas

3. The doctor has ordered the patient to be treated with drug C 0.8 mg. You have drug C 400 mcg/ml. How many ml do you administer?

4. The physician has ordered the patient be treated with drug D 150 mg. You have available to you 125 mg/tsp of the medication. How many ml do you administer?

5. The physician has ordered drug E gr 1/200. Available is drug E 0.3 mg per tablet. How many tablets do you administer?

6. The physician has ordered drug F 0.5 g. You find that you have 250 mg/5 ml of the medication. How much do you administer?

7. The doctor has ordered drug G 7.5 mg. You have 5-mg tablets on hand. How many tablets do you give?

8. You have an order for drug H 0.1 g. You have 50-mg tablets on hand. How many do you administer?

9. Drug J comes in a liquid that contains 500 mg/tbsp. You have an order for 125 mg. How many ml do you give?

10. The order is for drug K 0.05 g by injection and you have an ampule that reads "100 mg per ml." How many ml do you inject?

11. A vial of drug L labeled 1,200,000 units in 3 ml is available. How many ml are required to give the patient 600,000 units?

12. Drug M tablets gr 1⁄2 are available. How many tablets are required to administer 15 mg?

13. You are to give 0.2 g of a certain drug from a solution marked 50 mg in 1 ml. How many ml must you give?

Answers:

1. 1.5 tablets
2. 2 ml
3. 2 ml
4. 6 ml
5. 1 tablet
6. 10 ml
7. 1.5 tablets
8. 2 tablets
9. 3.75 ml
10. 0.5 ml
11. 1.5 ml
12. 1⁄2 tablet
13. 4 ml

From Math for Meds, (Curren, 2008)

When preparing a dosage of a powdered medication, be certain to read the package insert closely. It usually will give instructions on what type and how much of a diluent to use to convert the powder to a liquid form. *Never* try to substitute a liquid for the ordered diluent.

Dimensional Analysis

Dimensional analysis is a method of calculating dosages and solutions used in an effort to further reduce medication errors. It provides one method for calculating all types of drug problems. Dimensional analysis can most easily be understood by reviewing it as a step-by-step process.

Problem: The physician has ordered drug A 1,500 mg by mouth. On hand are tablets containing 500 mg of medication.

Step 1: Determine the label needed for the final answer to the problem. In this case it is tablets.

Step 2: Draw a grid to use in calculating the problem. It should be formatted as

$$? \text{ tab} = \frac{\quad\quad}{\quad\quad} \Bigg|$$

Step 3: Find a factor in the problem that has the same label as the final answer label. Insert that factor directly to the right and in the numerator position of the grid.

$$? \text{ tab} = \frac{1 \text{ tab}}{\quad\quad} \Bigg|$$

Step 4: Write the numbers in the problem that will show the existence of an accurate relationship. In this case the problem tells us that 1 tablet equals 500 mg of the medication.

$$? \text{ tab} = \frac{1 \text{ tab}}{500 \text{ mg}} \Bigg|$$

Step 5: Look at the label of the factor in the denominator position. In this case the label is milligrams. Find a factor in the problem that uses the same label and insert it into the upper right numerator position.

$$? \text{ tab} = \frac{1 \text{ tab}}{500 \text{ mg}} \Bigg| \; 1{,}500 \text{ mg}$$

Step 6: Cancel out the unit labels.

$$? \text{ tab} = \frac{1 \text{ tab}}{500 \text{ mg}} \bigg| \frac{1{,}500 \text{ mg}}{}$$

Step 7: Calculate using the information that is remaining.

$$? \text{ tab} = \frac{1 \text{ tab}}{500 \text{ mg}} \bigg| \frac{1{,}500 \text{ mg}}{} = 3 \text{ tablets}$$

Dimensional analysis can be adapted for use with problems that require conversion between units as well (Edmunds, 2006).

Calculate the following problems using dimensional analysis as the method of calculation.

1. You receive a physician's order for 1 mg of drug B. You have available 0.5 mg per tablet. Calculate the number of tablets to prepare.

2. You receive a physician's order for 0.6 g of drug C. You have available 300 mg per tablet. Calculate the number of tablets to prepare.

3. You receive a physician's order for 60 mg of drug D. You have available 15 mg per tablet. Calculate the number of tablets to prepare.

4. You receive a physician's order for 0.5 g of drug E. You have available 250 mg per 5 ml. Calculate the number of milliliters of medication to prepare.

5. You receive a physician's order for 125 mg of drug F. You have available 62.5 mg per 5 ml. Calculate the number of milliliters of medication to prepare.

6. You receive a physician's order for 75 mg of drug G. You have available 125 mg per 2 ml. Calculate the number of milliliters of medication to prepare.

Answers:

1. 2 tablets
2. 2 tablets
3. 4 tablets
4. 10 ml
5. 10 ml
6. 1.2 ml

From Edmunds (2006)

Calculation Involving Intravenous Infusions

Although hospitals routinely use electronic infusion pumps for instillation of intravenous (IV) fluids, it is imperative that the registered nurse is capable of calculating the infusion rate without the benefit of the electronic pump in the event of equipment failure. The nurse should be able to calculate the flow rate for administration of IV fluids as well as calculating the total amount of time needed to administer a specific infusion. When calculating the flow rate for administration of IV fluids, the nurse must be aware of both the flow rate and the drop factor. The *flow rate* is the rate at which IV fluids are given, and it is measured in drops per minute. The *drop factor* is the number of drops per milliliter of liquid and is determined by the size of the drops. The drop factor varies among manufacturers and is available on the infusion set's packaging. Usually, infusion sets have a drop factor of 10 or 15 drops/ml.

The formula for calculating the flow rate for an IV is

$$\text{drop factor} \times \text{milliliters/minute} = \text{flow rate (drops/minute)}$$

Problem: The physician orders the IV at 2 ml/min. The IV infusion set delivers 10 drops/ml. Calculate the flow rate of the IV.

$$10 \text{ drop/ml} \times 2 \text{ ml/min} = 20 \text{ drops/min}$$

Remember that if the physician orders the IV to infuse in ml/hr, convert the hour to 60 minutes. Occasionally, physicians' orders specify the time frame for an IV infusion. The nurse also may need to anticipate when a specially prepared bag of IV fluid needs to be replaced. To calculate the infusion time, the registered nurse will first need to calculate the flow rate.

The formula for calculating the total infusion time is

$$\frac{\text{Total drops to be infused} \times 60 \text{ (drops/hr)}}{\text{Flow rate (drops/min)}} = \text{total infusion time (hr and min)}$$

Problem: The physician orders 1,000 ml 0.9% normal saline to be infused at 50 drops/min. The drop factor for the infusion is 10 drops/ml. Calculate the infusion time for the IV.

$$1,000 \text{ ml} \times 10 \text{ drops/ml} = 10,000 \text{ drops}$$

$$\frac{10,000 \text{ drops}}{3,000 \text{ drops/hr}} = 3.33 \text{ hr or 3 hours and } 60 (.33) = 19.8 = 20 \text{ minutes}$$

When calculating the IV flow rate, it is impossible to measure a fraction of a drop, so round any partial drops to the nearest whole drop. When calculating infusion time, the time must be in hours and minutes. Remember to round to the nearest whole minute. When rounding, remember the rule of 0–4, round down; 5–9, round up.

Calculate the following IV flow rates using the correct formula.

1. The physician has ordered an IV to infuse at 75 ml/hr. How many gtt per minute do you give if the tubing delivered 60 gtt/ml?
2. The physician has ordered an IV to infuse at 125 ml/hr. How many gtt per minute do you give if the tubing delivered 15 gtt/ml?
3. The physician has ordered an IV to infuse at 150 ml/hr. How many gtt per minute do you give if the tubing delivered 20 gtt/ml?
4. The physician has ordered an IV to infuse at 80 ml/hr. How many gtt per minute do you give if the tubing delivered 10 gtt/ml?
5. The physician has ordered an IV to infuse at 150 ml/hr. How many gtt per minute do you give if the tubing delivered 15 gtt/ml?

Answers:

1. 75 gtt
2. 31 gtt
3. 50 gtt
4. 13 gtt
5. 38 gtt

Calculations Involving Infants and Children

Because of their small body weight and heightened sensitivity to medications, infants and children usually require special reduced dosages of medication to ensure they do not experience adverse reactions or undue side effects. Some medications will be ordered in terms of the child's body weight. *Clark's rule* can be used as a calculation aid in a case such as this. This uses the adult dosage of the medication and the weight of the child. The formula is written as

$$\frac{\text{weight of child}}{\text{weight of adult}} \times \text{adult dose} = \text{child's dose}$$

Consider the following example to see how Clark's rule could be used:

If the adult dosage of a medication is 100 mg, what is the dose for a 50-pound child (Edmunds, 2006)?

$$\frac{50 \text{ pounds}}{150 \text{ pounds}} \times 100 \text{ mg} = \frac{5,000}{150} = 33 \text{ mg}$$

Some medications are ordered with the dosage based on the age of the infant or child. *Young's rule* and *Fried's rule* can be useful in such a case. Young's rule is used for children ages 2 to 12, whereas Fried's rule is used for infants and small children under the age of 2. In the case of Young's rule the formula is

$$\frac{\text{child's age}}{\text{child's age} + 12} \times \text{adult dose} = \text{child's dose}$$

Consider this example to see how Young's rule could be used for a calculation:

If the adult dose of a medication is 0.5 g, what is the dose for an 8-year-old child?

$$\frac{8 \text{ yr}}{20} \times 0.5 \text{ g} = \frac{4}{20} = 0.2 \text{ g}$$

In the case of Fried's rule, the formula is

$$\frac{\text{infant's age in months}}{150} \times \text{adult dose} = \text{infant's dose}$$

Consider the example to see how Fried's rule could be used for a calculation:

If the adult dose of a medication is 1,000 mg, what is the dosage for a 3-month-old infant?

$$\frac{3 \text{ months} \times 1,000 \text{ mg}}{150} = \frac{3,000 \text{ mg}}{150} = 20 \text{ mg}$$

Summary of Key Points in Chapter

The chapter provided a review of the concepts required for calculation of dosages and solutions, such as

<   Use of ratio and proportion method of calculation
<   Use of desired over available method of calculation
<   Use of dimensional analysis method of calculation

< Use of formulas for calculation of intravenous flow rates as well as infusion times
< Use of formulas used in calculation of dosages for children:
  < Clark's rule
  < Fried's rule
  < Young's rule

Conclusion

Multiple types of dosage and solution calculations can be used during the course of a registered nurse's daily practice setting, and this chapter has in no way been intended to include all of them. However, it is the responsibility of the nurse to familiarize himself or herself with the formulas needed to calculate any type of dosage problem that could arise clinically.

Calculating dosages and flow rates of infusions is only one of the many roles the registered nurse may be called on to assume during the course of his or her career. The various roles of the registered nurse are discussed in the next chapter.

Critical Thinking Questions

1. Explain the ratio and proportion method of calculating dosages and solutions to a nursing student.
2. Explain the desired over available method of calculating dosages and solutions to a nursing student.
3. Explain the dimensional analysis method of calculating dosages and solutions to a nursing student.

Scenarios

1. The physician has ordered drug A 150 mg twice daily. On hand is drug A 75-mg tablets. How much do you give per dose?
2. The physician has ordered drug B 1.5 g. On hand is drug B 2 g in 5 ml. How many ml do you give per dose?
3. Order is for drug C 30 g. Drug C 30 g/15 ml is available. How many ml do you give per dose?
4. Drug D 10 mg by mouth is ordered for allergies. Drug D 5-mg tablets are available. How many tablets do you give per dose?
5. Order: drug E 6 mg by mouth q8h x3 doses. The available drug reads: drug E 4 mg/5 ml oral suspension. How many ml do you give per dose?

6. Order: Drug F 650 mg by mouth as needed for a temperature > 101°. On hand: 325-mg tablets. How much do you give per dose?

7. Order: Drug G 100 mg by mouth every 12 hours. On hand: Drug G 125 mg/5 ml. How much is administered per dose?

8. Drug H 150 mg is ordered. Available is 75 mg/7.5 ml. How many ml do you give?

9. Order: Drug J 50 mg every 4 hours as needed for pain. Drug J is supplied in 75 mg/1.5 ml. How much do you administer per dose?

10. The physician's order reads: Drug K 2.5 mg by mouth. The available drug reads: Drug K 5-mg scored tablets. How much do you administer?

11. The physician's order reads: Drug L 4 g by mouth daily. The available drug reads: Drug L 4-g tablets. How much do you administer?

12. The patient is receiving 750 mg of drug M four times daily. The label indicates drug M 250 mg/5 ml. Calculate amount of each dose.

13. Order: Drug N 0.125 mg by mouth daily. On hand: Drug N 0.25-mg tablets. How many do you administer?

14. Order reads: Drug P 8 mg by mouth daily. On hand: 5 mg/5 ml of drug P. How much do you give per dose?

15. Drug Q 0.6 g is ordered; available tablets contain 600 mg. How many tablets do you give per dose?

16. Drug R 2 g has been ordered every 12 hours. The available tablets are 500 mg each. What amount do you give per dose?

17. Drug S 75 mg is ordered; available tablets contain 25 mg. How many tablets do you give?

18. The patient is receiving 500 mg of drug T. The label indicates 250 mg/5 ml. Calculate the dose.

19. Drug U 300 mg is ordered. Available is 100 mg/1 ml. How many ml do you give?

20. Drug V 8,000 units SQ is ordered. On hand is 10,000 units per ml. How much do you give?

Answers:

1. 2 tablets
2. 3.8 ml
3. 15 ml
4. 2 tablets
5. 7.5 ml
6. 2 tablets
7. 4 ml

8. 15 ml
9. 1 ml
10. 0.5 or 1⁄2 tablet
11. 1 tablet
12. 15 ml
13. 0.5 or 1⁄2 tablet
14. 8 ml
15. 1 tablet
16. 4 tablets
17. 3 tablets
18. 10 ml
19. 3 ml
20. 0.8 ml

(From Cornett & Blume, 1991)

NCLEX® Questions

Using the information you obtained from studying this chapter, go online to complete the following NCLEX®-format review questions. Visit http://go.jblearning.com/terryLPN using the access code in the front cover of your book. This interactive resource allows you to answer each question and instantly review your results. Practice until you can answer at least 75% successfully, and then try to improve your score with each successive attempt.

1. Your patient has been ordered 100 mcg of drug A by mouth. The hospital pharmacy currently has available drug A in 25-mcg tablets. How many tablets do you give to administer the correct dosage?

2. Your patient has been ordered 250 mg of drug B by mouth. The hospital pharmacy currently has 100 mg per scored tablet. How many tablets do you give to administer the correct dosage?

3. Your patient needs 50 mg of drug C by mouth. You have on hand a bottle with a label that reads "drug C 12.5 mg/5 ml." How many ml do you give to administer the correct dosage?

4. Your patient is a 250-pound adult male. How many kilograms does he weigh? (Round your answer to the nearest hundredth.)

5. The patient has been ordered 240-mg suppositories of drug E. Available are suppositories with 120 mg of medication in each one. How many should be administered?

6. Your patient has an order for drug F 250 mg. The medication arrives from the hospital pharmacy as an oral suspension of 125 mg/5 ml. How many ml do you give to administer the correct dosage?

7. The physician orders your patient to receive drug G 75 mg. Your floor stocks a vial of the medication that contains 100 mg/ml. How many ml do you give to administer the correct dosage? (Round your answer to the nearest tenth.)

8. A patient has been ordered 0.25 mg of drug H. How many grams of this medication does this patient receive?

9. The patient has been ordered to receive 2 grains of a drug. The bottle is labeled 120 mg/ml. How many milliliters do you administer?

10. The physician ordered drug Q 5 mg by mouth for your patient. The medication is supplied as 2.5 mg of medication per tablet. How many tablets do you give to administer the correct dosage?

For more information on the topics in this chapter and others, please see Appendix on p. 299 for a list of web links to additional resources.

References

Burke, A. (2005). Calculation of dosages and solutions: Ratio and proportion. Retrieved from http://www.nurseceusonline.com/viewcourse/20-67010-p .htm

Cornett, E., & Blume, D. (1991). *Dosages and solutions: A programmed approach to meds and math.* Philadelphia, PA: F.A. Davis.

Curren, A. (2008). *Math for Meds: Dosages and solutions.* Florence, KY: Delmar.

Diehl, L. (2010). Brush up on your drug calculation skills. Retrieved from http://www.nursesaregreat.com

Edmunds, M. (2006). *Introduction to clinical pharmacology.* St. Louis, MO: Elsevier.

For a full suite of assignments and additional learning activities, use the access code located in the front of your book to visit this exclusive website: http://go.jblearning.com/terryLPN. If you do not have an access code, you can obtain one at the site.

CHAPTER OBJECTIVES

At the end of this chapter, you will be able to:

1. Describe the concept of reality shock and how it can affect the new graduate registered nurse.

2. Describe the various aspects of the registered nurse functioning as a preceptor.

3. Describe the various aspects of the registered nurse functioning as a researcher.

4. Describe the various aspects of the registered nurse functioning as a manager.

5. Describe the various aspects of the registered nurse functioning as an advocate.

6. Describe the various aspects of the registered nurse functioning as an educator.

KEY TERMS

case presentations
clinical trials
honeymoon phase
modeling

nurse advocate
observation
preceptor
reality shock

recovery phase
shock and rejection phase
whistle-blower
workplace advocate

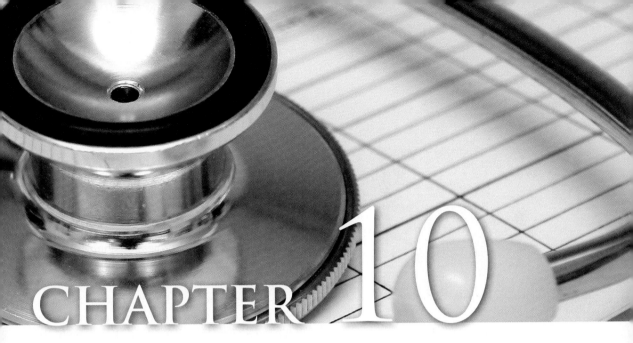

CHAPTER 10

Roles of the Registered Nurse

Introduction

The modern healthcare environment grows more complex and more technical on a daily basis, thus requiring the registered nurse (RN) to be more prepared than ever before to assume a variety of roles in the healthcare facility and to exercise both critical thinking and nursing judgment. The RN may be called on during the course of a single workday to act as an advocate, educator, manager, and researcher.

Transitioning into New Roles

Many professionals who enter the workforce after completing an educational program experience *reality shock*. This occurs when the new employee moves from the clearly defined role of the student into the more nebulous role of professional, in this case, the RN. Although the licensed practical nurse (LPN)-to-RN student is already familiar with the healthcare environment in many ways, he or she can still expect to experience reality shock to some degree as the "LPN" role is almost instantly shed and the new "RN" role is just as rapidly assumed.

Reality shock as it applies to nursing occurs in several phases (Zerwekh & Garneau, 2012):

< *Honeymoon phase*: The new RN is overjoyed to finally complete his or her educational program and begin working. A regular paycheck is

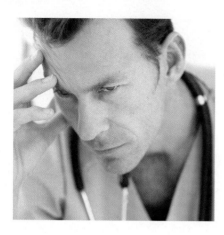

arriving, the stress of class work has been relieved, and all indications are that life is moving into an adventuresome but interesting new phase.

< *Shock and rejection phase*: In this phase the new RN begins to recognize a conflict existing between what was taught in the nursing program and what is actually occurring in the healthcare facility in daily practice. Some RNs may choose to reject the values learned in school and compromise their professional integrity by embracing the normal pattern of functioning in their work settings, whether that pattern yields high quality patient care or not. Other new RNs may experience a decrease in their self-esteem because they believe they are not fulfilling their new role adequately. Occasionally, the new RN will become angry and frustrated at their inability to fit into their newly assumed role and reject nursing as the right profession for them.

< *Recovery phase*: The new RN begins to transition into the new role by evaluating the work environment objectively and predicting how staff members usually will act in certain situations, such as when a family member is unhappy with a patient's care. This transition occurs by using several tools on the first day of the new job as an RN: setting priorities during the course of the workday, managing conflict effectively, managing time efficiently, and choosing a support group. The mere act of choosing a support of one's own making can be empowering for the new RN. The group should be composed of the nurse's preceptor during new employee orientation, other new LPN-to-RN graduates as well as other types of new RN graduates (Associate degree-to-Bachelor's degree and diploma-to- Associate degree-to-Bachelor's degree) and mentors that are both realistic and encouraging. Humor is also valuable to the new RN in that it can be used to resolve conflicts in a positive way; this acts as a boost to the new RN's self-esteem in the work setting. Finally, the new RNs who make the most successful transition recognize the existence of problems in their new work environments and work to make changes to produce higher quality patient care. Such changes, however small, serve as confidence boosters for the new RN.

Information about reality shock and its effect on the new RN will be valuable to the RN who is rapidly assuming a leadership role because of his or her previous work experience as an LPN. The nurse who has previously been an LPN and gained a wealth of work experience and now serves as a mentor to new, perhaps younger, RNs should bear in mind that work schedules are closely linked to job satisfaction. The new RN who is immediately thrust into working 12-hour nights may find it difficult to make the transition from the freedom of an academic schedule. Experienced nurses should have patience with the new graduate RN who complains about the frequency with which he or she works weekends, night shift, or holidays. The new employee's preceptor or mentor should review the RN's schedule to determine if he or she has been placed into a particularly grueling rotating day/ night schedule, for example. Offer advice on how to sleep during the day or how to work with a particularly difficult physician. Such assistance may help the new RN find his or her foothold as a nurse and may help the nursing unit avoid losing a potentially valuable employee (Halfer & Graf, 2006).

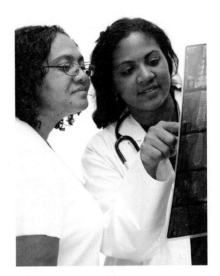

Role of the Nurse as Preceptor

As an experienced RN you may be called on to function in the role of a *preceptor*. A preceptor is an experienced RN who has proven his or her competence in nursing through performance in the work setting. Often, the preceptor works with senior-level nursing students during the last semester of their nursing program. The preceptor will be responsible for observing the student's performance, offering guidance when needed, and evaluating the student's ability to perform clinically as well as use critical thinking to manage a group of patients (Zerwekh & Garneau, 2012).

The RN can learn to function in the role of a preceptor in several ways. Initially, he or she must acquire an understanding of the adult learner, because the typical senior-level nursing student will be 21 or older. This type of learner is interested in blending his or her role as a senior-level nursing student with any previous roles acquired through life experience. Clinical activities should include both new experiences and previously acquired skills so the adult learner is continuously integrating those previous experiences with current skills. Also, because the adult learner who is a nursing student typically is experience focused, he or she will prefer to take an active part in the learning process. The student will benefit if the topic is of immediate value to him or her.

In addition, the preceptor, after considering how the adult learner will perform in the role of a nursing student, should consider where the student is located in the nursing program. This will tell the preceptor if the student needs a very structured approach, such as the first-year student in his or her first clinical setting, or much more autonomy, such as the student poised to graduate. The preceptor should recognize whether the adult student may become anxious in a situation requiring a significant amount of autonomy; conversely, the student may become frustrated if he or she has a large amount of experience with a situation that requires the student to be closely supervised (Burns, Beauchesne, Ryan-Krause, & Sawin, 2006).

To appropriately function as a preceptor in the clinical setting, Burns et al. (2006) suggested the preceptor be familiar with some basic principles of adult learning:

< Just as participation is known to be particularly important for the adult learner, repetition and reinforcement are also important to strengthen the learning that is occurring and to promote retention of the new content being absorbed.

< Varying the types of learning activities used can maintain a high level of learner interest and increase use of both new information and newly acquired skills; sufficiently prepare and plan settings for learning and clinical experiences to ensure minimal disruption to patient needs and expectations while still achieving the student's goals.

< Use various types of teaching strategies, including modeling, observation, case presentations, and direct questioning

< Understand how to appropriately evaluate the student's clinical learning experience; the preceptor should familiarize him- or herself with the curriculum of the student's nursing program, the goals and objectives for the student's clinical experience, and the type of tool used for evaluation of the student. Review the student's personal goals for the clinical experience, which should be realistic and yet more detailed than "to obtain a passing grade." Plan to have a session midway through the semester preceptorship so students can have ample time to make changes in their performance if needed. Notify the faculty member any time there are concerns raised about the student's performance.

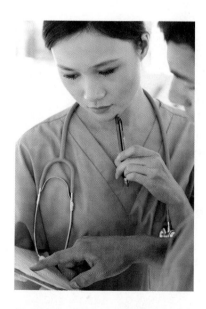

Functioning as a preceptor includes being able to use various types of teaching strategies. *Modeling* is used when the preceptor demonstrates clinical expertise while caring for patients as the nursing student observes. A significant part of modeling is *observation*, which allows the student to watch as the preceptor interacts with patients, problem solves using critical thinking and nursing judgment, and moves through the nursing process. Observation and modeling allow the student and preceptor to work together through the intricacies of various aspects of patient care.

Case presentations may be helpful in teaching the nursing student how to complete patient histories, develop nursing diagnoses, and interpret laboratory findings.

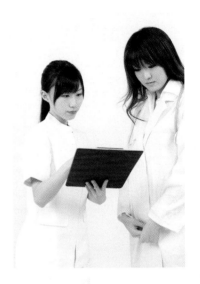

Different teaching strategies may foster the development of critical thinking in the student. Direct questioning can be used along with a calm manner to encourage the student to state why he or she believes a certain thing is relevant to a patient. Neher, Gordon, Meyer, and Stevens (1992) described a method, "the one minute preceptor method," to be easily used in the clinical setting. This method consists of six steps:

1. Obtain a commitment from the student: This is accomplished by asking questions such as "What lab work should be drawn on this patient?" and "What medications should this patient receive?"

2. Seek out supporting evidence for the commitment: The student should be able to explain why he or she believes certain tests should be run or certain medications ordered.

3. Reinforce the student's success: Commend the student for correctly identifying tests to be run, medications that are appropriate, or noting specific assessment findings.

4. Offer guidance on the student's errors: Review sections the student omitted or incorrectly assessed.

5. Teach a general principle: If the student incorrectly identified or failed to identify assessment findings because a basic principle was missed, the preceptor may need to review, for example, how pediatric vital signs differ from adult vital signs.

6. Conclude the session: State the next action on the part of the preceptor and the student. This could consist of instructing the student to monitor the patient's vital signs every hour for the next 4 hours so the student and the preceptor can evaluate the blood pressure trends (Neher, Gordon, Meyer, & Stevens, 1992).

Finally, the preceptor should provide instruction based on the developmental level of the student. There are three basic developmental levels of students, each one with its own knowledge base and skill set. The beginner usually needs the support of the preceptor in every area of the clinical learning experience. He or she probably has had minimal experience with patients and may be struggling with moving from being an expert in his or her previous field to being a novice in nursing. With this student the preceptor will probably need to use observation to assess the student's clinical skills. The second level is the transitional learner. With this learner the preceptor will need to give the student space enough to use more clinical reasoning. This student is able to provide more effective and efficient nursing care and thus will need to be assigned more complex patients. Case presentations are an effective teaching strategy with this type of learner. Finally, the preceptor will work with the competent proficient learner. This student is able to compare his or her current clinical experience with past experiences and thus is comfortable with the preceptor being less directly involved with clinical supervision. The student will recognize his or her limitations, ask questions, and seek out interaction with more knowledgeable clinicians. Frequently, the preceptor will derive a great deal of professional satisfaction from working with a student who has progressed from the level of beginner to that of proficient learner and subsequent colleague (Burns et al., 2006).

Role of the Nurse as Researcher

The RN who takes a position in full-time research plays a valuable role in the conduction of clinical trials in the field of oncology. *Clinical trials* are the various testing phases for new drugs used in the treatment of cancer patients, and they are required to be conducted under very strict conditions because of the use of actual patients during the testing. Although this is not the only way in which an RN can function in the role of full-time researcher, it is quite frequently seen in areas having large teaching hospitals.

Because the RN who serves as a full-time researcher frequently works with actual patients during the course of the research project, such as occurs with cancer clinical trials, he or she must have an exhaustive knowledge of the protocols that govern the research. Time may be of the essence when working with patients in the final stages of a terminal illness, and the researcher must have as much information as possible committed to memory to avoid wasting time searching for specific guidelines on a drug (Mais, 2006).

The RN functioning in the role of researcher will not be strictly confined to use of a computer but rather must ensure that he or she has hands-on clinical skills that are every bit as honed as they were when the nurse was functioning as a bedside clinician. For example, the RN assisting in the conduction of clinical trials with cancer patients may be called on frequently to start an intravenous access with a patient, and because of the caustic nature of chemotherapeutic drugs, the access must be virtually perfect to avoid the possibility of any of the drug seeping out of the vein and into the patient's surrounding tissues. Also, because these drugs often have the tendency to cause an anaphylactic response (severe allergic reaction), the RN may find it helpful to become certified in advanced cardiac life support in the event of a patient requiring resuscitation (Mais, 2006).

In addition, the nurse researcher must also have well-honed writing skills. Because the research team has the joint goals of prolonging patients' life spans and strengthening the quality of their lives as well as publishing the research findings in an attempt to assist patients globally, every step of the process must be carefully documented in detail. Every response of every patient must be described minutely; every scrap of information obtained on a blood sample must be recorded without omission because that omitted data could save a patient's life. The RN must assess and reassess patients persistently to detect any change that occurs in response to the medication, whether for better or worse. Omitted information could result in the research project being refused for publication, thus making the entire endeavor useless because the findings could not be used (Mais, 2006).

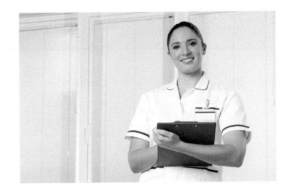

Finally, the RN as full-time researcher has a tremendous obligation to educate multiple people throughout the entire course of the research project: the patients who volunteer to be involved, the nurses who are caring for the patients, the family members concerned about how well the new medications will work, and even members of the community who need to be informed about the new drugs that may soon be available to help fight the scourge of cancer. The patients who volunteer to participate in the clinical trials need to be educated initially to determine if they are prepared both mentally and physically to participate. The education process should continue throughout the clinical trial to enable the patient to stop the trial and remove him- or herself if need be. The nurses trained to implement the clinical trial protocol will need almost constant education on the changes they can expect to see in patients after use of the drug as well as changes that are out of the ordinary. In this way the nurse can recognize if the patient is experiencing an adverse reaction to the drug. The patients' family members should receive frequent education on changes that may be expected in the patient's condition after treatment with the drug. Providing the family with information helps alleviate their anxiety, which in turn helps the patient feel more secure. Finally, the education of the public is a requirement to help build a base of support for the research team that may assist in future funding and to bring attention to the lives that are being saved as a result of such medical research (Mais, 2006). It is through the work of the nurse researcher who is part of an overall research team that evidence-based nursing practice continues to advance year by year.

Table 10-1 offers a comparison of the roles of nurse preceptor and nurse researcher.

TABLE 10-1 Comparison of the Roles of Nurse Preceptor and Nurse Researcher

Role	Definition	Functioning in the Role
Nurse Preceptor	A *preceptor* is considered to be an experienced RN who has proven his or her competence in nursing through performance in the work setting.	Typically, the preceptor will work with senior-level nursing students during their last semester of their nursing program. The preceptor will be responsible for observing the student's performance, offering guidance when it is needed, and evaluating the student's ability to perform clinically as well as use critical thinking to manage a group of patients. The preceptor may utilize some variation on the "One Minute Preceptor Method": 1. obtain a commitment from the student 2. seek out supporting evidence for the commitment 3. reinforce the student's success 4. offer guidance on the student's errors 5. teach a general principle 6. conclude the session
Nurse Researcher	The registered nurse who serves as a *nurse researcher* typically works with actual patients in the conduction of clinical trials. The *clinical trials* are the various testing phases for new drugs used in the treatment of cancer patients, and they are required to be conducted under very strict conditions because of the use of actual patients during the testing.	Because the RN who serves as a full-time researcher will be frequently working with actual patients during the course of the research project, he or she must have an exhaustive knowledge of the protocols that govern the research. The RN who is functioning in the role of researcher will not be strictly confined to use of a computer, but rather must ensure that he or she has hands-on clinical skills that are every bit as honed as they were when the nurse was functioning as a bedside clinician. The nurse researcher must not only have excellent clinical skills and knowledge of the protocols being utilized, but must only have well-honed writing skills.

Role of the Nurse as Manager

The RN may be called on to function in the role of manager at some point in his or her nursing career. The nurse manager is not necessarily synonymous with the nurse leader, because a leader generally chooses to assume that role and a manager is most often selected for the role and then appointed to the position. Marquis and Huston (2012) described nurse managers as follows:

< Have a position specially assigned to them within the organization
< Have delegated authority accompanying their position that provides them with a legitimate source of power
< Are expected to carry out certain duties and responsibilities that have been entrusted to them
< Are specifically concerned with maintaining control, making decisions, and analyzing the decision process as it occurs and the results of that process
< Manipulate employees, the workplace setting, fiscal resources, time, and other available resources to attain the goals set in conjunction with the facility's mission and vision
< Have a greater responsibility and accountability for rational decision-making and day-to-day control assigned by the formal organization than that assigned to the nurse leader
< Are capable of directing subordinate employees, whether they are easily led or are directed with difficulty

The manager actually functions to provide direction to any group that is working toward accomplishing a common goal. Usually, the manager strives to accomplish four things:

< Plan what needs to be done
< Organize how this activity is to be accomplished
< Direct who is to implement the activity
< Control when it is to be carried out and in what manner

Planning is the most basic and time consuming of these functions. It begins with the development of goals that reflect the organization's mission and vision and the development of strategies designed to accomplish the goals. Planning will continue as the manager decides on the requirements needed to accomplish the work and how to make those materials or personnel available. The manager must also design a contingency plan to cope with unexpected occurrences that could prevent the strategies from being accomplished. The nurse manager will use the same type of planning skills used as a staff nurse to accomplish the daily plan of care of each assigned patient (Zerwekh & Garneau, 2012).

In the organization phase the nurse manager matches the work to be accomplished with the resources available to implement the project. The nurse manager will need to have all information available on the work to be accomplished and the qualifications of the personnel available to fulfill the task. For example, if the work to be accomplished is to renovate the medication room of the nursing unit so the nurses can prepare medications more efficiently and effectively, the nurse manager will need to know the following information (Zerwekh & Garneau, 2012):

- The budget for the renovation
- What types of new equipment and material can be purchased
- What equipment is outdated and needs to be discarded
- What equipment and material needs to be upgraded to a different model or manufacturer because the current model or manufacturer is ineffective
- Availability of personnel such as carpenters and painters who could be pulled from other renovations in the hospital to assist with the medication room project, and the availability of another space close by to use as a medication room while the current one is undergoing renovation.

The manager must direct personnel, being accountable for verifying work is completed according to schedule and in accordance with applicable standards and the policies and procedures of the facility. Part of directing and supervising personnel involves the manager recognizing when patient care fails to meet applicable standards or begins to fall below the established quality assurance measures for the nursing unit. When this occurs the manager is responsible for ensuring action is taken to guarantee the safety and overall well-being of patients and that the performance of the staff who allowed the quality of patient care to deteriorate is addressed. If staff are found to require a maximum amount of supervision and direction to achieve the minimal compliance with standards, the manager must determine why they do not respond to his or her efforts to motivate them (Zerwekh & Garneau, 2012).

The manager will need to be aware of all types of regulations that will affect patient care and the overall functioning of the nursing unit. These can include the standards imposed by The Joint Commission as well as the regulations unique to the Centers for Medicare and Medicaid Services. A vital part of the control function of the nurse manager is being able to convey these regulations and standards to staff members in such a way that they can comprehend them easily and be able to comply with them (Zerwekh & Garneau, 2012).

Role of the Nurse Advocate

The RN is required by the American Nurses' Association's Code of Ethics to act as a patient advocate. The nurse must be prepared to defend a patient's decision even when the nurse doesn't agree with it and even if the nurse is the only supporter of the patient's choice. Essentially, the *nurse advocate* acts to protect patients from being abused and having their rights violated. The advocate is responsible for providing the patient with information he or she needs to make informed decisions about health care. This may involve the nurse consulting with an attorney or a religious leader of the patient's choice to gain the information needed to assist the patient. The RN is specially equipped to serve as a patient advocate because of the complex knowledge base of the nurse. The patient requires the nurse's knowledge of the modern healthcare system to navigate his or her way through the maze of physicians, diagnoses, laboratory findings, Medicare and Medicaid issues, and insurance reimbursements. In addition, the nurse is specially equipped to serve as a patient advocate because of the nurse–patient relationship. The nurse is privy to information about the patient that may not be available to any other member of the healthcare team and as such usually has proven his or her ability to maintain patient confidentiality regarding information such as patient coping styles, substance abuse, and mental illness (Wilkinson & Treas, 2011).

A variation on the role of the nurse advocate is the *workplace advocate*. The nurse manager ensures the work environment is safe for employees to work in and also is supportive of their growth both personally and professionally. Subordinate employees can expect a nurse manager who functions as a workplace advocate to

< Give them schedules that are reasonable and possible
< Keep overtime to a minimum
< Maintain staffing ratios at the level needed to promote safe patient care
< Pay wages comparable with those paid by similar hospitals in the area
< Allow nurses a part in the overall governance of the unit by participating in unit conferences.

Another form of nurse advocate is the *whistle-blower*. This is the nurse who brings the wrong-doing of an organization to the attention of the public. Whistle-blowing may be internal or external, occurring within an organization or by individuals outside of the facility. It requires great courage on the part of the advocate, because frequently the whistle-blower is ostracized by other employees who fear getting caught up in the unfolding scandal. Many employees fear retaliation and thus will avoid whistle-blowing, even though as nurses we have an obligation to report substandard practice (Marquis & Huston, 2012).

Finally, the RN must not only be an advocate for the patient but for the profession of nursing. The nurse should participate in the American political process and attempt to influence policymakers so that nursing has a say in issues that affect the healthcare delivery system. Also, legislators can be provided with copies of research studies so they can be positively influenced by evidence to make decisions favoring nursing and health care. Legislators and other policymakers are usually more willing to dialogue with large groups of nurses rather than individuals. RNs who join national nursing professional associations and specialty organizations automatically are more positively able to influence health care in America (Marquis & Huston, 2012).

Traditionally, nurses have shied away from becoming politically active advocates for the profession of nursing, preferring instead to advocate solely at the grassroots level of the individual patient. In the modern age of health care, with its multiple legal and ethical issues, problems with reimbursement of insurance carriers, and the complicating factor of the national debt, RNs must be prepared to advocate at all levels of the profession: not only at the level of the individual patient but also nationwide for the American nursing profession and potentially even globally through involvement in international nursing organizations (Marquis & Huston, 2012).

Role of the Nurse Educator

As the nursing shortage persists despite multiple stopgap measures, the need continues for large numbers of additional nurse educators to train new nurses in basic nursing programs and to serve in healthcare facilities to provide instruction to nurses on clinical and professional issues. Many RNs stated the following as factors that influenced their pursuit of a career as a nurse educator (Penn, Wilson, & Rosseter, 2008):

‹ Opportunity to influence the next generation of nurses
‹ Ability to share clinical expertise

< Opportunity to influence student success
< Ability to model professional values and clinical skills
< Ability to influence quality of health care delivered by future nurses

Initially, the RN should determine what type of position he or she is interested in pursuing. This could range from a full-time position teaching in a BSN program in a 4-year university to an adjunct position as a clinical instructor in an ADN or LPN program. Such a decision may lead the RN to pursue additional education, because teaching in a BSN program usually requires a doctoral degree. Furthermore, choosing to pursue a position as a clinical instructor requires maintaining clinical proficiency in the nurse's chosen area of practice. RNs who are interested in continuing a clinical focus to their career yet would also like to pursue a doctoral degree now have the option of attaining the Doctor of Nursing Practice. This degree is considered an alternative to the traditional PhD that involves completion of a lengthy research project and the writing of a dissertation. The degree of Doctor of Nursing Practice, by alternative, involves a clinically focused research project that is much less lengthy and no dissertation. Many RNs start their teaching career as a clinical adjunct to begin gaining experience in interacting with students, assuming the instructor role in a hospital setting, and learning how to accurately evaluate students at the clinical level (Penn et al., 2008).

The RN who is considering pursuing a career in education should begin building a curriculum vita (CV). This is essentially a resume tailored to the academic environment. The CV is a comprehensive list of all professional experiences, such as courses taught, presentations given, committee memberships obtained, research conducted, and awards received. Whereas the typical business-related resume now is expected to be 1 to 2 pages, the CV for a faculty member with several years of experience could be 20 pages or more (Penn et al., 2008).

The most effective teachers of adult learners, such as those in a nursing program, are those who encourage students to ask questions, find meaning in their queries, and apply new information. The modern nurse educator must be able to work with multiple generations of nurses who are present in the nursing workforce and be creative and innovative enough to make learning interesting and exciting for each one of them.

Whereas the 18-year-old nursing student might prefer an online assignment simply because it prevents the student from being required to go to class, the 45-year-old nursing student might prefer an online assignment because it gives him or her additional hours to work at a part-time job to support a family. In addition, the modern nurse educator must be technologically savvy enough to help a student download appropriate clinical applications for his or her personal data assistant while also maintaining the clinical competence to demonstrate a new skill for the student to observe. The educator's ultimate goal is to promote the development of clinical judgment and critical thinking in the student through the use of evidence-based practice.

Table 10-2 compares the roles of nurse manager, nurse advocate, and nurse educator.

TABLE 10-2 **Comparison of the Roles of Nurse Manager, Nurse Advocate, and Nurse Educator**

Role	Definition	Functioning in the Role
Nurse manager	The *nurse manager* is not necessarily synonymous with the nurse leader, since a leader generally chooses to assume that role, and a manager is most often selected for the role and then appointed to the position.	Managers typically: ‹ have a position specially assigned to them within the organization ‹ have delegated authority accompanying their position that provides them with a legitimate source of power ‹ are expected to carry out certain duties and responsibilities that have been entrusted to them ‹ are specifically concerned with maintaining control, making decisions, analyzing the decision process as it occurs, and the results of that process ‹ manipulating employees, the workplace setting, fiscal resources, time, and other available resources to attain the goals that have been set in conjunction with the facility's mission and vision ‹ have a greater responsibility and accountability for rational decision-making and day-to-day control assigned by the formal organization than that assigned to the nurse leader, and ‹ be capable of directing subordinate employees. ‹ The manager strives to accomplish four things: plan what needs to be done, organize how this activity is to be accomplished, direct who is to implement the activity, and control when it is to be carried out and in what manner.

Role	Definition	Functioning in the Role
Nurse advocate	The *nurse advocate* acts to protect patients from being abused and having their rights violated.	The registered nurse is required by the American Nurses' Association's Code of Ethics to act as a patient advocate. This means that the nurse is prepared to defend a patient's decision even when the nurse doesn't agree with it and even if the nurse is the only supporter of the patient's choice. The advocate is responsible for providing the patient with information he or she needs to make informed decisions about his/her health care. A variation on the role of the nurse advocate is the workplace advocate. This means that the nurse manager ensures that the work environment is safe for employees to work in and also is supportive of their growth both personally and professionally. Another form of nurse advocate is the whistle-blower. This is the nurse who brings the wrong-doing that is occurring in an organization to the attention of the public. Finally, the registered nurse must not only be an advocate for the patient but for the profession of nursing.
Nurse educator	The *nurse educator* both trains new nurses in basic nursing programs as well as serves in healthcare facilities to provide instruction to nurses on clinical as well as professional issues.	Many RNs have stated that some of the factors that influenced their pursuit of a career as a nurse educator included: ‹ opportunity to influence the next generation of nurses ‹ ability to share clinical expertise ‹ opportunity to influence student success ‹ ability to model professional values and clinical skills ‹ ability to influence quality of health care delivered by future nurses. ‹ The RN should determine what type of position he or she is interested in pursuing. This could range from a full-time position teaching in a BSN program in a four-year university to an adjunct position as a clinical instructor in a ADN or LPN program. Such a decision will also lead the RN to decide on the need to pursue additional education, since the desire to teach in a BSN program will usually require the acquisition of a doctoral degree. Furthermore, choosing to pursue a position as a clinical instructor will require maintaining clinical proficiency in the nurse's chosen area of practice. The RN who is considering pursuing a career in the role of nurse educator should begin building a curriculum vita (CV).

Summary of Key Points in Chapter

The chapter discussed the various roles of the RN, including that of preceptor, researcher, manager, advocate, and educator. The various stages of reality shock that the new graduate RN may experience as he or she transitions into the practice role of the bedside nurse also was discussed. The chapter included topics such as

‹ Characteristics of an effective preceptor
‹ Skills necessary to function as a nurse researcher
‹ Functions of a nurse manager
‹ Nurse functioning as a patient advocate, workplace advocate, whistle-blower, and advocate for the profession of nursing
‹ Motivating factors that would lead an RN to become a nurse educator

Conclusion

The profession of registered nursing is unique in its ability to allow a practitioner to serve in multiple roles over the course of a lifetime career, whether as a preceptor, a manager, a researcher, an advocate, or an educator, in addition to functioning as a bedside nurse. The practitioner who can serve in multiple roles throughout his or her career not only derives the satisfaction of developing a multifaceted career portfolio but also makes a remarkable contribution to healthcare delivery on potentially the national or even global level. The educator uses evidence-based practice to help nursing students develop clinical judgment and critical thinking. Evidence-based practice is discussed in the next chapter.

Critical Thinking Questions

1. Describe the reality shock you experienced when you first assumed the role of LPN in a healthcare facility. What did you do to cope with the reality shock?
2. Think about the first preceptor you ever had as an LPN. Was this person helpful to you and effective in the role of preceptor? Why or why not?

3. If you have functioned in the role of preceptor previously, which teaching strategies did you use? Were they effective for working with that student? If you have never served as a preceptor, which teaching strategies do you believe would most fit with your current work environment?

4. Think about the first nurse manager you ever had as an LPN. Was this person helpful to you and effective in the role of manager? Why or why not? What qualities distinguished the most effective nurse manager with which you ever worked?

5. Think of a nurse manager you know is not effective in that role. How does the staff that works under this individual usually function on a daily basis?

6. Consider your current work environment. If you were asked to assume the position of nurse manager today in that area, consider how you would carry out the functions of
   < Planning
   < Organizing
   < Directing or supervising
   < Controlling

7. Consider how you could function as an advocate
   < At the local level with individual patients
   < At the national level for the American nursing profession
   < Globally for the nursing profession
   Describe how your involvement at each of these levels could allow you to function as an advocate.

Scenarios

1. You are mentoring a new graduate RN who is experiencing reality shock. What can you do to help him as he begins to assume the role of RN?

2. Do you believe a full-time nurse researcher would be a useful addition in the facility where you are employed? Why or why not? Can you think of ways in which the work of a nurse researcher could be used on a unit that works with critically ill pediatrics patients?

3. You are an assistant nurse manager who is assigned to work with a nurse manager who cannot carry out the functions of a manager (planning, organizing, directing, and controlling). What can you do to cope with this situation?

4. You are an associate-degree prepared RN who is considering pursuing the role of a nurse educator. Document all the steps you might need to implement to achieve this.

NCLEX® Questions

Using the information you obtained from studying this chapter, go online to complete the following NCLEX®-format review questions. Visit http://go.jblearning.com/terryLPN using the access code in the front cover of your book. This interactive resource allows you to answer each question and instantly review your results. Practice until you can answer at least 75% successfully, and then try to improve your score with each successive attempt.

1. The RN is functioning as a preceptor and assists the nursing student in learning how to complete patient histories, develop nursing diagnoses, and interpret laboratory findings. The preceptor is most likely to be using
   a. modeling
   b. observation
   c. case presentations
   d. direct questioning

2. The RN is functioning as a preceptor. She is most likely to encourage the student to state why he believes a certain thing is relevant to the student's patient by using
   a. modeling
   b. observation
   c. case presentations
   d. direct questioning

3. The RN is functioning as a preceptor. She allows the nursing student to watch as the preceptor starts an IV. The preceptor is using
   a. modeling
   b. mentoring
   c. case presentations
   d. direct questioning

4. The nurse preceptor obtains a commitment from the nursing student on an assessment and determines the student's supporting evidence for

the commitment. According to the "one minute preceptor method," the next step for the preceptor is to

a. conclude the session

b. teach a general principle

c. reinforce the student's success

d. offer guidance on the student's errors

5. The nurse preceptor offers guidance on the student's errors. According to the "one minute preceptor method" the next action on the part of the preceptor is to

a. conclude the session

b. teach a general principle

c. reinforce the student's success

d. offer guidance on the student's errors

6. The new graduate RN obtains his first job and is relieved to have the security of a steady paycheck. This phase of reality shock as the role of RN is being assumed is most likely to be

a. recovery phase

b. shock phase

c. rejection phase

d. honeymoon phase

7. The RN who acts to protect patients from being abused and having their rights violated is most aptly described as functioning as a

a. workplace advocate

b. preceptor

c. nurse advocate

d. mentor

8. The nurse manager goes to nursing administration to ask for the funds needed to send three nurses for additional training to allow them to get national certifications. This nurse is functioning as a

a. workplace advocate

b. preceptor

c. nurse advocate

d. mentor

9. Joe is an RN with 10 years' experience who consistently demonstrates his expertise in patient care as well as his professionalism toward his coworkers on a daily basis. This qualifies Joe to be considered as a:

a. workplace advocate

      b. preceptor

      c. nurse advocate

      d. mentor

10. Sue is a nurse manager who requests that the unit have new lighting installed because it is inadequate for the nurses to work in. This qualifies Sue to be considered as a

11. workplace advocate

12. preceptor

13. nurse advocate

14. mentor

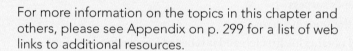
For more information on the topics in this chapter and others, please see Appendix on p. 299 for a list of web links to additional resources.

References

Burns, C., Beauchesne, M., Ryan-Krause, P., & Sawin, K. (2006). Mastering the preceptor role: Challenges of clinical teaching. *Journal of Pediatric Health Care, 20*, 172–183.

Halfer, D., & Graf, E. (2006). Graduate nurse perceptions of the work experience. *Nursing Economics, 24*, 150–155.

Mais, K. (2006). The role of the research nurse in hospital based oncology clinical trials. *Oncology News, 1*, 22–23.

Marquis, B. L., & Huston, C. J. (2012). *Leadership roles and management functions in nursing* (7th ed.). Philadelphia, PA: Lippincott Williams & Wilkins.

Neher, J., Gordon, K., Meyer, B., & Stevens, N. (1992). A five-step "microskills" model of clinical teaching. *Journal of the American Board of Family Practice, 5*, 419–424.

Penn, B., Wilson, L., & Rosseter, R. (2008) Transitioning from nursing practice to a teaching role. *OJIN: Online Journal of Issues in Nursing, 13*. Retrieved from http://www.nursingworld.org/MainMenuCategories/ANAMarket place/ANAPeriodicals/OJIN/TableofContents/vol132008/No3Sept08 /NursingPracticetoNursingEducation.aspx

Wilkinson, J., & Treas, L. (2011). *Fundamentals of nursing* (2nd ed.). Philadelphia, PA: F.A. Davis.

Zerwekh, J., & Garneau, A. (2012). *Nursing today: Transitions and trends* (7th ed.). St. Louis, MO: Elsevier.

For a full suite of assignments and additional learning activities, use the access code located in the front of your book to visit this exclusive website: http://go. jblearning.com/terryLPN. If you do not have an access code, you can obtain one at the site.

At the end of this chapter, you will be able to:

1. Describe the basic process of implementing evidence-based practice.

2. Describe the ACE star model of evidence-based practice.

3. Describe the Iowa model of evidence-based practice.

4. Discuss the "PICO" method of framing a clinical question.

5. Discuss the classifications for clinical questions.

ACE star model
discovery
evaluation

evidence-based practice
evidence summary
implementation

Iowa model
translation

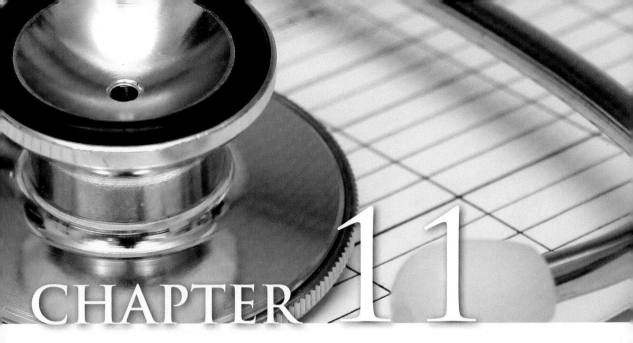

CHAPTER 11

Evidence-Based Practice

Introduction

As health care continues to change in response to new advances and modern technology, nurses are increasingly called on to integrate evidence-based practice into their daily patient care. Although many definitions exist, the one that may best capture the essence of *evidence-based practice* (EBP) is that it is the consistent use of research-based information to make decisions that will affect patient care delivery. To correctly use evidence in nursing practice, the registered nurse must use critical thinking to review research, evaluate its relevance to nursing as a profession, and then decide if it can be used in healthcare delivery (Schmidt & Brown, 2009). The best evidence in the form of research along with the nurse's own clinical expertise and the patient's values and preferences are used together to make clinical decisions, increase the chance of optimal clinical outcomes, and enhance the overall patient quality of life (Schardt & Mayer, 2010).

Implementing Evidence-Based Practice

Once the registered nurse understands what EBP is and the importance of using it correctly, the nurse should review the step-by-step process of how EBP is implemented. It consists of several stages (Schardt & Mayer, 2010):

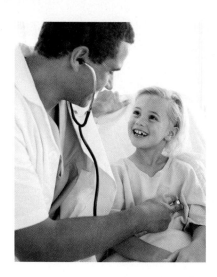

< Assess the patient: Consider a clinical problem that has arisen from caring for the patient. An appropriately worded clinical question should include four elements:

  < Patient and the patient's problem: Consider how such a patient would be described. What is his or her main problem, disease process, or condition? Is gender, age, or race relevant to the diagnosis or the treatment plan?

  < Intervention or action being considered: This is the action the nurse is considering implementing, such as tests to be ordered or instruction on medication to be given, or a factor that is influencing the patient's current situation, such as age or use of recreational drugs.

  < Comparison between the chosen intervention and the primary alternative: This could consist of deciding between two different medications or two different diagnostic tests. Be aware that all interventions do not require a comparison.

  < Outcomes the nurse hopes to accomplish, measure, improve, or otherwise affect: Essentially, this is what the nurse is trying to do for the patient, such as relieving pain or improving mobility.

< Ask the question: Develop a well-constructed clinical question based on the clinical problem. Carefully consider the type of question asked and type of evidence of greatest concern. Typically, questions related to clinical tasks are classified as

  < Diagnosis: The question may be concerned with how to choose and interpret various diagnostic tests.

  < Therapy: The question may be concerned with how to choose a treatment regimen for the patient.

  < Prognosis: The question may be concerned with how to evaluate the patient's clinical progression and anticipate complications.

  < Harm/etiology: The question may be concerned with how to identify causes of a disease process.

< Acquire the evidence: Choose the appropriate resources to use as evidence and conduct a search to extract the information. These could consist of summaries of the primary evidence available, databases, electronic textbooks, as well as meta-search engines that may allow a nurse to obtain the highest quality clinical evidence rapidly.

< Appraise the evidence: Evaluate the evidence gathered for validity (is it rooted in truth?) and applicability (is it useful in clinical practice or is it so esoteric as to not be helpful?).

< Apply: Integrate the evidence that has proven to be helpful into clinical experience and patient preferences and apply it to healthcare delivery.

< Self-evaluate: The nurse should evaluate his or her own performance with the patient.

Iowa Model of Evidence-Based Practice

The Iowa model of evidence-based practice is a method of understanding how research must be considered within the entire healthcare system to guide practice decisions. Developed at the University of Iowa, the model emphasizes the importance of considering the healthcare provider, the patient, and the facility infrastructure as evidence gathered is incorporated into nursing practice. According to the Iowa model, the process of incorporating evidence-based practice should occur according to the following stages:

< Identify a "trigger" that is either problem focused or knowledge focused and will demonstrate the need for change to occur. A problem-focused trigger could consist of a clinical problem or a new risk management issue, whereas a knowledge-focused trigger could consist of new research or new practice guidelines. In choosing a trigger consider the magnitude of the problem (is it widespread?), its applicability (is it applicable to all areas of practice in the healthcare facility?), its likelihood of being able to improve care, the availability of research on the topic, and the commitment of healthcare staff to change in this area (Doody & Doody, 2011).

< Determine if the trigger issue is a priority for the healthcare organization; if it is not a priority for the organization but only for the healthcare provider, it will probably not be an effective trigger. For the trigger to be considered as an intervention, it should be effective in the entire healthcare organization and supported by administration.

< Doody and Doody (2011) suggested that a team should be formed at this point to develop the question involving the trigger issue, to be responsible for the implementation of the proposed change in practice, and then to evaluate the results of the change. Also, at this point factors that can interfere with incorporating research findings into practice should be addressed, such as workload, level of education of staff, lack of support from management and colleagues,

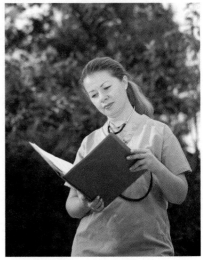

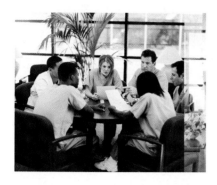

lack of exposure to the process of performing research, and availability of time.

< Frame the clinical question so an accurate literature search can occur. Develop the question using the "PICO" formula:
  < P = The patient population
  < I = The area of interest under consideration or the potential intervention that could be implemented
  < C = The intervention used for comparison purposes or the control group of patients being used
  < O = The outcome that is being sought as a result of the proposed change in practice
< Review and evaluate relevant evidence and determine if there is sufficient evidence to warrant a change in nursing practice. Also determine if the research studies being reviewed are appropriate for use with the patient population available to the nurse researcher in the facility's clinical setting.
< Identify the evidence that will support the change in clinical practice.
< Implement the change in practice (Dontje, 2007).

Table 11-1 provides a comparison between the basic process of implementing EBP and the Iowa model.

TABLE 11-1 Comparison of Basic Process of Implementing Evidence-Based Practice and the Iowa Model of Evidence-Based Practice

Basic Process of Implementing Evidence-Based Practice	Iowa Model of Evidence-Based Practice
Assess the patient—Consider a clinical problem that has arisen from caring for the patient.	Identify a "trigger" that is either problem focused or knowledge focused and will demonstrate the need for change to occur; a problem-focused trigger could consist of a clinical problem that has been discovered, or a new risk management issue that has developed, whereas a knowledge-focused trigger

Basic Process of Implementing Evidence-Based Practice	Iowa Model of Evidence-Based Practice
	could consist of new research that has been released or new practice guidelines that have been developed. Determine if the "trigger" issue that has been identified is a priority issue for the healthcare organization; if it is not a priority for the organization, but only for the healthcare provider, it will probably not be an effective trigger; if the trigger is an intervention that is being considered, it should be one that would be effective in the entire healthcare organization and would be supported by administration.
Ask the question—Develop a well-constructed clinical question based on the clinical problem. An appropriately worded clinical question should include four elements: P = the patient and the patient's problem—Consider how such a patient would be described. What is his main problem, disease process, or condition? Is his gender, or race relevant to the diagnosis or the treatment plan? I = the intervention or action being considered. This is the action that the nurse is considering implementing, such as tests to be ordered or instruction on medication to be given, or a factor that is influencing the patient's current situation, such as age, or use of recreational drugs. C = comparison between the chosen intervention and the primary alternative. This could consist of deciding between two different medications or two different diagnostic tests. Be aware that all interventions do not require a comparison. O = outcomes that the nurse hopes to accomplish, measure, improve, or otherwise affect. Essentially, this is what the nurse is trying to do for the patient, such as relieving pain or improving mobility.	Frame the clinical question so that an accurate literature search can occur; develop the question suing the "PICO" formula: P = the patient population I = the area of interest under consideration or the potential intervention that could be implemented C = the intervention used for comparison purposes or the control group of patients being utilized O = the outcome that is being sought as a result of the proposed change in practice

Basic Process of Implementing Evidence-Based Practice	Iowa Model of Evidence-Based Practice
Carefully consider the type of question being asked and type of evidence of greatest concern. Typically, questions related to clinical tasks are classified as: diagnosis—the question may be concerned with how to choose and interpret various diagnostic tests therapy—the question may be concerned with how to choose a treatment regimen for the patient prognosis—the question may be concerned with how to evaluate the patient's clinical progression and anticipate complications harm/etiology—the question may be concerned with how to identify causes of a disease process.	
Acquire the evidence—Choose the appropriate resources to use as evidence and conduct a search to extract the information. These could consist of summaries of the primary evidence available, databases, electronic textbooks, as well as meta-search engines that may allow a nurse to obtain the highest quality clinical evidence rapidly.	Review and evaluate relevant evidence and determine if there is sufficient evidence to warrant a change in nursing practice; also determine if the research studies being review are appropriate for utilizing with the patient population available to the nurse researcher in the facility's clinical setting.
Appraise the evidence—Evaluate the evidence that has been gathered for validity (is it rooted in truth?) and applicability (is it useful in clinical practice, or is it so esoteric as to not be helpful?).	Identify the evidence that will support the change in clinical practice.
Apply—Integrate the evidence that has proven to be helpful into clinical experience and patient preferences and apply it to healthcare delivery. Self-evaluate—The nurse should evaluate his or her own performance with the patient.	Implement the change in practice

Source: Schardt & Mayer, 2010; Dontje, 2007.

ACE Star Model

The *ACE star model*, another model helpful in understanding EBP, provides a framework within which to organize the various concepts included in EBP as they progress toward knowledge transformation. The points of the "star" correspond to the following stages (Melnyk & Fineout-Overholt, 2005):

< *Discovery*: In this stage new knowledge is being produced by research methods used in original research studies.
< *Evidence summary*: Evidence from all research studies available is combined so that the nurse researcher has the current scientific view of the topic.
< *Translation*: Clinical recommendations are generated that are both valid and reliable and are the result of evidence summaries combined with clinical expertise. By the conclusion of this stage, knowledge now reflects best practice and is based on evidence, consensus, and the endorsement of experts in the field. In this stage a healthcare agency may choose to adopt practice guidelines that are specific to a certain patient population.
< *Implementation*: Evidence influences clinical decision-making and begins to change nursing practice. Effective implementation cannot occur without considering efficiency (is it efficient to use in terms of cost, personnel, and time?), currency (is it timely for the patient population under consideration?), and usefulness (is it something that will be readily used by both the client and the nurse?).
< *Evaluation*: The effectiveness of the change in nursing practice should be evaluated by the patient population, the healthcare provider, and the overall healthcare system.

Table **11-2** compares the models of EBP.

TABLE 11-2 Comparison of Models of Evidence-Based Practice

Basic Process of Implementing Evidence-Based Practice	Iowa Model of Evidence-Based Practice	ACE Star Model
Assess the patient—Consider a clinical problem that has arisen from caring for the patient.	**Identify** a "trigger" that is either problem focused or knowledge focused and will demonstrate the need for change to occur; a problem-focused trigger could consist	**Discovery**—This is the stage of the model when new knowledge is being produced by research methods used in original research studies.

Basic Process of Implementing Evidence-Based Practice	Iowa Model of Evidence-Based Practice	ACE Star Model
	of a clinical problem that has been discovered, or a new risk management issue that has developed, whereas a knowledge-focused trigger could consist of new research that has been released or new practice guidelines that have been developed. Determine if the "trigger" issue that has been identified is a priority issue for the healthcare organization; if it is not a priority for the organization, but only for the healthcare provider, it will probably not be an effective trigger; if the trigger is an intervention that is being considered, it should be one that would be effective in the entire healthcare organization and would be supported by administration.	
Ask the question—Develop a well-constructed clinical question based on the clinical problem. An appropriately worded clinical question should include four elements: P = the patient and the patient's problem—Consider how such a patient would be described. What is his main problem, disease process, or condition? Is his gender or race relevant to the diagnosis or the treatment plan?	**Frame** the clinical question so that an accurate literature search can occur; develop the question using the "PICO" formula: P = the patient population I = the area of interest under consideration or the potential intervention that could be implemented	

Basic Process of Implementing Evidence-Based Practice	Iowa Model of Evidence-Based Practice	ACE Star Model
I = the intervention or action being considered. This is the action that the nurse is considering implementing, such as tests to be ordered or instruction on medication to be given, or a factor that is influencing the patient's current situation, such as age, or use of recreational drugs.	C = the intervention used for comparison purposes or the control group of patients being utilized O = the outcome that is being sought as a result of the proposed change in practice	
C = comparison between the chosen intervention and the primary alternative. This could consist of deciding between two different medications or two different diagnostic tests. Be aware that all interventions do not require a comparison.		
O = outcomes that the nurse hopes to accomplish, measure, improve, or otherwise affect. Essentially, this is what the nurse is trying to do for the patient, such as relieving pain or improving mobility.		
Carefully consider the type of question being asked and type of evidence of greatest concern. Typically, questions related to clinical tasks are classified as: diagnosis—the question may be concerned with how to choose and interpret diagnostic tests		

Basic Process of Implementing Evidence-Based Practice	Iowa Model of Evidence-Based Practice	ACE Star Model
therapy—the question may be concerned with how to choose a treatment regimen for the patient prognosis—the question may be concerned with how to evaluate the patient's clinical progression and anticipate complications harm/etiology—the question may be concerned with how to identify causes of a disease process.		
Acquire the evidence—Choose the appropriate resources to use as evidence and conduct a search to extract the information. These could consist of summaries of the primary evidence available, databases, electronic textbooks, as well as meta-search engines that may allow a nurse to obtain the highest quality clinical evidence rapidly.	**Review and evaluate** relevant evidence and determine if there is sufficient evidence to warrant a change in nursing practice; also determine if the research studies being review are appropriate for utilizing with the patient population available to the nurse researcher in the facility's clinical setting.	**Evidence summary**—evidence from all research studies available is combined so that the nurse researcher has the current scientific view of the topic. **Translation**—clinical recommendations are generated that are both valid and reliable and are the result of evidence summaries combined with clinical expertise. By the conclusion of this stage, knowledge now reflects best practice and is based on evidence, consensus, and the endorsement of experts in the field. This is the stage when a healthcare agency may choose to adopt practice guidelines that are specific to a certain patient population.

Basic Process of Implementing Evidence-Based Practice	Iowa Model of Evidence-Based Practice	ACE Star Model
Appraise the evidence—Evaluate the evidence that has been gathered for validity (is it rooted in truth?) and applicability (is it useful in clinical practice, or is it so esoteric as to not be helpful?).	Identify the evidence that will support the change in clinical practice.	
Apply—Integrate the evidence that has proven to be helpful into clinical experience and patient preferences and apply it to healthcare delivery. Self-evaluate—The nurse should evaluate his or her own performance with the patient.	**Implement** the change in practice	**Implementation**—evidence influences clinical decision-making and begins to change nursing practice. Effective implementation cannot occur without considering efficiency (is it efficient to utilize in terms of cost, personnel, and time?), currency (is it timely for the patient population under consideration?), and usefulness (is it something that will be readily used by both the client and the nurse?).
		Evaluation—the effectiveness of the change in nursing practice should be evaluated by the patient population, the healthcare provider, and the overall healthcare system.

Source: Schardt & Mayer, 2010; Dontje, 2007; Melnyk & Fineout-Overholt, 2005.

Assessing a Nursing Research Article

Once the topic of concern has been selected and the question has been designed, the nurse can begin selecting the evidence. To initially begin locating articles that might be helpful, the following databases usually yield a treasure trove of information:

CINAHL Plus
PubMed
PsycINFO
AssessMedicine
Cochrane Database of Systematic Reviews
Current Medical Diagnosis and Treatment
Academic Search Premier
Nursing and Allied Health
ERIC
JBI Connect
MEDLINE
Sage Premier
Scopus
Science Direct
EBSCOhost

However, it must be determined what is being sought as the nurse reviews each article being scrutinized. When reading a nursing research article as part of a literature search for evidence, there are specific areas of the article that should be reviewed to determine important pieces of information (Zerwekh & Garneau, 2012):

- *Problem statement, purpose, research question, result/findings* to determine if the overall content of the article is relevant to the question
- *Problem statement or literature review* to determine why the research was conducted
- *Date of publication* to determine if the research was current or if findings are outdated
- *Method and design sections* to determine what research method was used to conduct the study, the intended subjects of the study, the sample of participants used, and the setting in which the research was conducted

< *Findings and discussion* to determine if the findings will be useful to the nurse and the question that has been developed

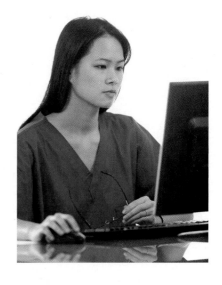

Implications of Evidence-Based Practice for the Registered Nurse

What are the greater implications of EBP for the registered nurse? For an intervention derived from evidence to involve all clinicians in a facility, nurse managers and ultimately the director of nursing must consider the cost of implementing the intervention, barriers that could slow the change process, facilitators that could cause the process of implementation proceed more smoothly, and the education that will be needed staff-wide for implementation to occur. All nurses have a responsibility as practitioners to both locate and use the research that other nurse researchers have already generated (Wilkinson & Treas, 2011).

Ultimately, nurses must overcome some basic obstacles that would prevent them from using research in everyday healthcare delivery (Wilkinson & Treas, 2011):

< Basic lack of knowledge of nursing research: Nurses must practice reviewing articles available on various databases to recognize which ones relate most closely to his or her field of practice.
< Negative feelings toward the research process: The research process can be a daunting challenge for any professional, but the registered nurse should not avoid reviewing research articles simply because of a lack of understanding of some aspects of the process. Negative feelings toward the research process can be overcome as the nurse reviews multiple articles on various databases to gain understanding.

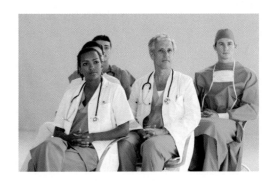

< Few avenues for research dissemination: Nurses may lack an understanding of research because they rarely hear it discussed by experts; this can be alleviated by nurses attending conferences where research findings are discussed and explained.

< Lack of support from the healthcare facility: Nurses may avoid reading research articles and attempting to incorporate evidence into daily practice because the healthcare facility does not make EBP a priority; however, the registered nurse can incorporate some evidence on his or her own as long as the interventions do not require a commitment of time or money from the facility. Making small changes in nursing practice in response to evidence can allow the nurse to serve as a role model to other nurses and encourage them to do the same.

< Study findings do not fit the clinical environment: Registered nurses may become discouraged when they review studies that do not seem to be applicable to their practice settings. This barrier can be eliminated by reviewing studies from multiple databases. Frequently, a clinician will find that studies from one specific database seem to most closely fit his or her practice settings.

Summary of Key Points in Chapter

Here we discussed the significance of EBP to the modern registered nurse. Various methods of describing the implementation of EBP were described, including the ACE star model and the Iowa model. In addition, the "PICO" method of framing a clinical question was described along with the classifications for clinical questions.

Conclusion

EBP is invaluable for the registered nurse because of the validity it provides to his or her practice as a clinician. The knowledge of a sound theoretical basis for every intervention pursued as a nurse provides confidence, a sense of community with other nurses, and pride in the profession that would see the necessity in EBP.

The evidence provided by research should be incorporate into every professional area of the nurse's life. It can be a gold mine of assistance when the RN is faced with the need for critical decisions. The decision-making process is discussed in the next chapter.

Critical Thinking Questions

1. You are caring for a 63-year-old Hispanic man diagnosed with congestive heart failure. Write a clinical question for this patient utilizing the elements of PICO.

   a. What type of question did you develop? Does it concern diagnosis, therapy, prognosis, or harm/etiology?

   b. Select at least three resources to use as evidence for this question and conduct a search for information.

   c. Evaluate the evidence you gathered. Is it valid? Is it applicable to your clinical practice?

   d. Decide how you would integrate the evidence into your current clinical practice.

   e. Do you believe your current clinical practice would change if you used the evidence gathered?

   f. How do you foresee using this evidence in your clinical practice when you become a registered nurse?

2. You are caring for a 25-year-old African American woman who is experiencing a sickle cell crisis. She is a single mother to a 2-year-old little boy. Write a clinical question for this patient using the elements of PICO.

   a. What type of question did you develop? Does it concern diagnosis, therapy, prognosis, or harm/etiology?

   b. Select at least three resources to use as evidence for this question and conduct a search for information.

   c. Evaluate the evidence you gathered. Is it valid? Is it applicable to your clinical practice?

   d. Decide how you would integrate the evidence into your current clinical practice.

   e. Do you believe your current clinical practice would change if you used the evidence gathered?

   f. How do you foresee using this evidence in your clinical practice when you become a registered nurse?

3. You are caring for a 12-year-old boy diagnosed with bladder cancer. His parents are in the midst of a bitter divorce. Write a clinical question for this patient using the elements of PICO.

   a. What type of question did you develop? Does it concern diagnosis, therapy, prognosis, or harm/etiology?

     b. Select at least three resources to use as evidence for this question and conduct a search for information.

     c. Evaluate the evidence you gathered. Is it valid? Is it applicable to your clinical practice?

     d. Decide how you would integrate the evidence into your current clinical practice.

     e. Do you believe your current clinical practice would change if you used the evidence gathered?

     f. How do you foresee using this evidence in your clinical practice when you become a registered nurse?

4. You are caring for a 15-year-old pregnant girl who came into the emergency department this afternoon in labor. Write a clinical question for this patient using the elements of PICO.

     a. What type of question did you develop? Does it concern diagnosis, therapy, prognosis, or harm/etiology?

     b. Select at least three resources to use as evidence for this question and conduct a search for information.

     c. Evaluate the evidence you gathered. Is it valid? Is it applicable to your clinical practice?

     d. Decide how you would integrate the evidence into your current clinical practice.

     e. Do you believe your current clinical practice would change if you used the evidence gathered?

     f. How do you foresee using this evidence in your clinical practice when you become a registered nurse?

5. You are caring for a 3-year-old Hispanic girl who was brought into the emergency department after she and her parents went through a tornado. Her parents have not yet been found. The child speaks only Spanish. Write a clinical question for this patient using the elements of PICO.

     a. What type of question did you develop? Does it concern diagnosis, therapy, prognosis, or harm/etiology?

     b. Select at least three resources to use as evidence for this question and conduct a search for information.

     c. Evaluate the evidence you gathered. Is it valid? Is it applicable to your clinical practice?

     d. Decide how you would integrate the evidence into your current clinical practice.

  e. Do you believe your current clinical practice would change if you used the evidence gathered?

  f. How do you foresee using this evidence in your clinical practice when you become a registered nurse?

6. Compare and contrast the basic process of implementing EBP and the Iowa model of EBP in your own words.

7. Compare and contrast the Iowa model of EBP and the ACE star model in your own words.

8. Compare and contrast the basic process of implementing EBP, the Iowa model of EBP, and the ACE star model in your own words.

Scenarios

You are considering using bullying behavior among nurses in the workplace as your topic of interest as you perform a literature search for evidence. Using this topic, consult the following databases for information:

CINAHL Plus
PubMed
PsycINFO
AssessMedicine
Cochrane Database of Systematic Reviews
Current Medical Diagnosis and Treatment
Academic Search Premier
Nursing and Allied Health
ERIC
JBI Connect
MEDLINE
Sage Premier
Scopus
Science Direct
EBSCOhost

Locate at least three articles and review the following sections of each one:

 < *Problem statement, purpose, research question, result/findings* to determine if the overall content of the article is relevant to the question

‹ *Problem statement or literature review* to determine why the research was conducted

‹ *Date of publication* to determine if the research was current or if findings are outdated

‹ *Method and design sections* to determine what research method was used to conduct the study, the intended subjects of the study, the sample of participants, and the setting in which the research was conducted

‹ *Findings and discussion* to determine if the findings will be useful to the nurse and the question developed

NCLEX® Questions

Using the information you obtained from studying this chapter, go online to complete the following NCLEX®-format review questions. Visit http://go.jblearning.com/terryLPN using the access code in the front cover of your book. This interactive resource allows you to answer each question and instantly review your results. Practice until you can answer at least 75% successfully, and then try to improve your score with each successive attempt.

1. The PICO stages are included in which step of implementation of evidence-based practice?
   a. asking the question
   b. assessing the patient
   c. acquiring the evidence
   d. appraising the evidence

2. The registered nurse is determining if evidence gathered is going to be useful in his clinical practice. This is most applicable to the _____ step of implementing evidence-based practice.
   a. asking the question
   b. assessing the patient
   c. acquiring the evidence
   d. appraising the evidence

3. The registered nurse decides the best resources to use as evidence and then conducts a search to generate the needed information. This is most applicable to the _____ step of implementing evidence-based practice.
   a. asking the question
   b. assessing the patient
   c. acquiring the evidence

d. appraising the evidence

4. The registered nurse notes the clinical question is concerned with how to identify the causes of a disease process. This clinical question is most likely to be classified as

   a. prognosis
   b. harm/etiology
   c. diagnosis
   d. therapy

5. The registered nurse notes the clinical question is concerned with choosing a treatment regimen for the patient. This clinical question is most likely to be classified as

   a. prognosis
   b. harm/etiology
   c. diagnosis
   d. therapy

6. The registered nurse notes the clinical question is concerned with interpreting the results of various diagnostic tests. This clinical question is most likely to be classified as

   a. prognosis
   b. harm/etiology
   c. diagnosis
   d. therapy

7. The registered nurse notes the clinical question is concerned with evaluating the patient's clinical progression. This clinical question is most likely to be classified as

   a. prognosis
   b. harm/etiology
   c. diagnosis
   d. therapy

8. The registered nurse is using the ACE star model to help understand evidence-based practice. The nurse generates clinical recommendations that are both valid and reliable. This corresponds to which stage of the model?

   a. implementation
   b. translation
   c. evidence summary
   d. discovery

9. The registered nurse is using the ACE star model to help understand evidence-based practice. The nurse locates new knowledge that is generated by research methods used in original research studies. This corresponds to which stage of the model?

   a. implementation

   b. translation

   c. evidence summary

   d. discovery

10. The registered nurse is using the ACE star model to help understand evidence-based practice. The nurse combines information from all research studies to get the current scientific view of the topic. This corresponds to which stage of the model?

    a. implementation

    b. translation

    c. evidence summary

    d. discovery

For more information on the topics in this chapter and others, please see Appendix on p. 299 for a list of web links to additional resources.

References

Dontje, K. (2007). Evidence-based practice: Understanding the process. *Topics in Advanced Practice Nursing eJournal, 7*. Retrieved from http://www.medscape.com/viewarticle/567786_4

Doody, C.M., & Doody, O. (2011). Introducing evidence into nursing practice: Using the IOWA model. *British Journal of Nursing, 20(11)*, 661–664.

Melnyk, B., & Fineout-Overholt, E. (2005). *Evidence-based practice in nursing & healthcare*. Philadelphia, PA: Lippincott Williams and Wilkins.

Schardt, C., & Mayer, J. (2010, July). Introduction to evidence-based practice. Retrieved from http://www.hsl.unc.edu/services/tutorials/ebm/welcome.htm

Schmidt, N., & Brown, J. (2009). *Evidence-based practice: Appraisal and application of research*. Sudbury, MA: Jones and Bartlett.

Wilkinson, J., & Treas, L. (2011). *Fundamentals of nursing* (2nd ed.). Philadelphia, PA: F.A. Davis.

Zerwekh, J., & Garneau, A. (2012). *Nursing today: Transitions and trends* (7th ed.). St. Louis, MO: Elsevier.

For a full suite of assignments and additional learning activities, use the access code located in the front of your book to visit this exclusive website: http://go. jblearning.com/terryLPN. If you do not have an access code, you can obtain one at the site.

WWW

CHAPTER OBJECTIVES

At the end of this chapter, you will be able to:

1. Describe basic steps in the decision-making process.
2. Discuss factors that could serve as obstacles to the decision-making process.
3. Discuss types of group decision-making.
4. Describe factors unique to the individual that could affect the decision-making process.
5. Discuss various types of tools that could assist in the decision-making process.

WWW

KEY TERMS

consensus building
critical thinking
decision-making
Delphi group technique
judgment

left-brain-dominant
   thinkers
nominal group technique
patient cue
problem solving

right-brain-dominant
   thinkers
scenario planning
trial and error

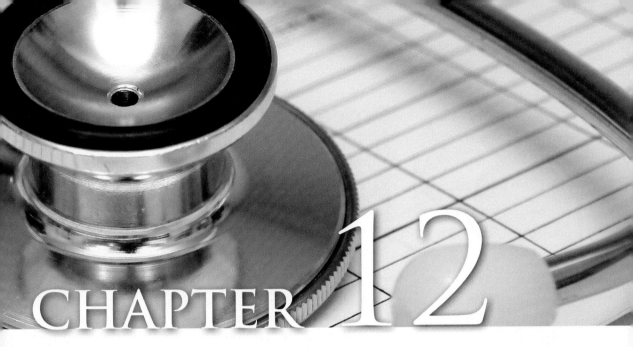

CHAPTER 12

Clinical Decision-Making as a Registered Nurse

Introduction

The registered nurse (RN) practicing in today's healthcare environment is bombarded with volumes of data about patients that must be constantly evaluated and processed mentally. For the data to be processed accurately, the RN must be capable of critical thinking and clinical judgment and of using a comprehensive knowledge base and a wide-ranging clinical skill set. The RN who can accurately process data will be able to make decisions.

Defining Decision-Making

Huber (2010) described decision-making as the essence of what the nurse leader and nurse manager are expected to do. The RN who makes decisions in haste or without accurately processing data can be the catalyst for life-threatening consequences for the patient. For all practical purposes, *decision-making* consists of choosing a certain course of action. Part of decision-making is *problem solving*, which involves analyzing a specific situation and identifying the course of a particular problem that led to the specific situation. Decision-making also relies greatly on critical thinking. *Critical thinking* involves the ability to examine the evidence provided, use reasoning to analyze it, and then develop a judgment about the evidence (Marquis & Huston, 2012).

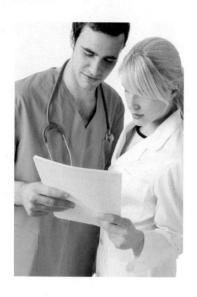

Process of Decision-Making

The RN's ability to engage in clinical decision-making is primarily derived from knowledge gained from the nursing profession, from his or her own internal stores of knowledge, and from information gained from the patient care situation. The clinical decision-making process begins when the RN recognizes a *patient cue*; this is either a specific response from the patient or the absence of a response that is appropriate for the specific patient situation. The cue will cause the RN to begin seeking out additional information about the situation. This information will lead to a *judgment*, which is the most definitive conclusion the RN can determine. Once that conclusion has been formed, the RN must then plan a course of action. That decision must ultimately be evaluated as to its effectiveness (Gillespie, 2010). Kelly (2010) summarized the basic steps in the decision-making process:

< Identify the need for a decision to be made
< Gather data about the situation
< Identify the key participants who will be affected by the decision
< Determine the desired outcome of the decision
< Identify all possible alternatives, along with the potential benefits and possible consequences of each alternative
< Make a decision based on all information available
< Follow through on the decision that has been made
< Evaluate the decision to determine its effectiveness

The progressive nature of the decision-making process is shown in **Figure 12-1**.

There are factors that could derail the RN who is on track to make an evidence-based decision. The following criteria could potentially act as obstacles to the decision-making process (Kelly, 2010):

< Past experiences
< Personal values
< Personal biases
< Preconceived ideas
< Drawing conclusions without thorough examination of the situation
< Failing to take the time to obtain all available information
< Selecting a decision that is too complicated to implement

FIGURE 12-1 The Decision-Making Process

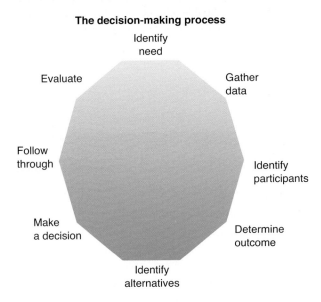

The decision-making process

Identify
need

Evaluate

Gather
data

Follow
through

Identify
participants

Make
a decision

Determine
outcome

Identify
alternatives

< Selecting a decision that is too widespread to implement
< Failing to communicate information about the decision that is selected to all involved participants
< Failing to evaluate the decision appropriately to assess its effectiveness.

Group Decision-Making

The decision-making process can change when the decision is made by a group. Specific decision-making techniques should be used by a group. The ***nominal group technique*** involves the group members initially writing out their ideas about the issue in question and then presenting those ideas to the other group members along with the potential benefits and drawbacks. The process then moves into an opportunity for the ideas to be clarified and evaluated, and, finally, group members will vote privately on the ideas presented (Kelly, 2010).

The second type of group technique is the ***Delphi group technique***, which uses questionnaires to obtain group members' opinions. The responses are summarized and then distributed to group members repeatedly until group consensus is achieved. Because this technique can be used with a large number of participants, it has the potential to generate a large number of ideas. Finally, *consensus building* by no means indicates that all group members are in complete agreement with all aspects of the decision made; however, it does mean that all group members are capable of being supportive of that decision (Kelly, 2010). **Table 12-1** compares the types of group decision-making.

TABLE 12-1 Comparison of the Types of Group Decision-Making

Types of Group Decision-Making	Tool(s) Used	Number of Participants	Steps in Process
Nominal	Group members write out their ideas	More effective with a smaller group	1. Group members write out their ideas about the issue in question, and then present those ideas to the other group members along with the potential benefits and the drawbacks. 2. There is an opportunity for the ideas to be clarified and evaluated. 3. Group members vote privately on the ideas presented.
Delphi	Uses questionnaires to obtain group members' opinions	Can be effectively used with a large group	1. Questionnaires are distributed to obtain group members' opinions. 2. Responses are summarized and then distributed to group members repeatedly until group consensus is achieved.
Consensus building	No formal tools to bring group members into agreement	No limit on the number of participants; however, the time required to achieve consensus may act as a limiting factor	Group members do not have to be in complete agreement with all aspects of the decision that has been made; however, it does mean that all group members are capable of being supportive of the decision that has been made.

Source: Kelly, 2010.

Role of the Individual in Decision-Making

The initial step in the decision-making process is identifying the need for a decision to be made. This involves the individual perceiving and evaluating the situation in a manner that is unique to him or her. Various individual aspects greatly influence the decision-making process (Marquis & Huston, 2012) (**Table 12-2**):

‹ Gender: Research has shown that frequently women may be more concerned about the consequences of a decision than men and also tend to be more concerned about any restrictions placed on them during the decision-making process. In comparison, men tend to be more concerned with analysis of the information needed to implement the decision as well as the goals of the decision (Missri, 2008).

‹ Values: The decision will ultimately be influenced by the values of the individual. The available alternatives and the one selected for the final decision are products of values. The person may consciously or unconsciously limit some of the alternatives because of his or her personal belief system. Values also influence how data are gathered and processed.

‹ Life experience: The more mature the level of the individual and the broader his or her life experiences, the more available alternatives there will be. Also, how much autonomy people seek influences how much decision-making experience they have already accumulated.

‹ Individual preference: When considering alternatives, the individual will consider risks that he or she considers to be particularly important, such as time and energy expenditures, financial risk, potential emotional trauma, and perceived physical risk.

‹ Thinking styles: Most people are believed to have dominance of either the right or left hemisphere of the brain. It is thought that analytical thinkers are left brain dominant, whereas creative or intuitive thinkers are right brain dominant. *Left-brain-dominant thinkers* typically excel at tasks that require use of language, logic, numbers, and anything that uses sequential ordering. In comparison, *right-brain-dominant thinkers* excel at tasks that require nonverbal ideas and those that pull concepts together into a whole structure. The left-brain-dominant individual will tend to do particularly well when focusing on mathematics, reading, planning, and organizing, whereas the right-brain-dominant individual will tend to do especially well concentrating on images, music, colors, and patterned items.

TABLE 12-2 Effect of Individual Factors on Decision-Making

Types of Factor	Description	Effect on Decision-Making Process
Gender	Women may be more concerned about the consequences of a decision than men are, and also tend to be more concerned about any restrictions that will be placed on them during the decision-making process; men tend to be more concerned with analysis of the information need to implement the decision as well as the goals of the decision	When the decision to be made could potentially have dire consequences (such as leading to a patient's death if the wrong decision is made), it may be helpful to have predominantly women on the committee making the decision; if there are specific goals attached to the decision, it will be helpful to have predominantly men on the committee because they will be more concerned with whether the goals are being fulfilled.
Values	The alternatives that are viewed as being available as well as the one that is selected for the final decision will be a product of values. The person may consciously or unconsciously limit some of the alternatives because of the personal belief system. Values will also influence how data is gathered as well as processed.	Recognize that having individuals on a decision-making committee who have strong convictions, moral views, and religious beliefs may lead to some limiting of alternatives but probably will lead to a decision being made that is congruent with the facility's mission statement.
Life experience	The more mature the level of the individual and the broader his or her life experiences, the more alternatives will be viewed as being available; also, since some people will seek autonomy more than others, this will influence how much decision-making experience they have already accumulated.	If the decision-making committee is made up of members with fairly narrow life experiences, it may tend to limit the number of alternatives available. Conversely, if the members have a broad spectrum of experiences, the number of alternatives may also be broadened. The process may proceed with difficulty if members have had little experience with the decision-making process.

Types of Factor	Description	Effect on Decision-Making Process
Individual preference	When considering alternatives, the individual will consider risks that he or she considers to be particularly important, such as time and energy expenditures, financial risk, potential emotional trauma, and perceived physical risk.	Individuals who are primarily concerned about potential risks in certain areas such as finances will tend to have difficulty agreeing to an alternative that encompasses financial risk, even if the other group members are accepting of it. Furthermore, a decision-making committee member may seem to take the possibility of risk in certain areas very lightly, such as disfavor in the community, when in reality the committee member simply does not personally consider this to be an area of major risk.
Thinking styles	Most people are believed to have dominance of either the right or left hemisphere of the brain. It is thought that analytical thinkers are left-brain-dominant while creative or intuitive thinkers are right-brain-dominant. **Left-brain-dominant thinkers** typically excel at tasks that require use of language, logic, numbers, as well as anything that utilizes sequential ordering. In comparison, **right-brain-dominant thinkers** excel at tasks that require nonverbal ideas as well as those that pull concepts together into a whole structure; the left-brain-dominant individual will tend to do particularly well when focusing on mathematics, reading, planning, and organizing, while the right-brain-dominant individual will tend to do especially well concentrating on images, music, colors, and patterned items.	If the committee must make a decision regarding finances, and it is made primarily of right-brain-dominant individuals, the process will probably be a difficult one. These individuals will not see this as being a priority and essentially will look at the "big picture." However, if such a committee is made up of primarily left-brain-dominant individuals, it also will be a difficult process because of the members will be concerned about finances and will be detail-oriented. A mixture of half right-brain-dominant and half left-brain-dominant would be ideal for the committee members.

Source: Marquis & Huston, 2012.

Tools to Aid the Decision-Making Process

Once the RN has a clear understanding of how the process of decision-making proceeds and the various factors that affect it, the actual mechanics of implementing the process must be set in motion. The RN can use various strategies when implementing the decision-making process:

- *Trial and error*: The RN selects a solution that seems to be a likely choice and tries it. The nurse manager who uses this as a consistent method of making decisions is perceived as ineffective and as having a poor grasp of evidence-based practice.
- Pilot projects: The RN tries a solution with a small number of participants as a limited trial. The pilot project allows the nurse to try a solution on a limited basis so that major problems can be detected early, thus minimizing risk.
- Creativity techniques: These can include brainstorming, the Delphi process, and nominal group techniques. These work particularly well with a complicated problem that has no clear-cut solution. The goal in this case is to generate potential solution without the encumbrance of possible bias.
- Decision tree: This model allows the nurse to visualize the alternatives available as well as various outcomes. Usually, a question is asked with various options that result in branching. For example, the decision tree shown in **Figure 12-2** asks, "Can a unit manager be hired for nursing unit by January 1st?" Depending on the answer to the problem, the corresponding path will be followed downward with the resulting consequences provided.
- *Scenario planning*: This group strategy works well with situations that change frequently. It asks the question "what if?" and therefore allows for the development of a wide variety of possible outcomes. Such scenarios can serve to illuminate areas of potential development as well as risk for a facility.
- Worst-case scenario: This is particularly useful when considering decisions that involve risk. The scenario technique progresses to the point of having everything that possibly could go wrong culminate in disaster simultaneously. This allows alternatives with their potential consequences to be ranked as "most desirable" and "least desirable." It also allows a facility to foreshadow the possible long-range effects of implementing a certain decision (Huber, 2010).

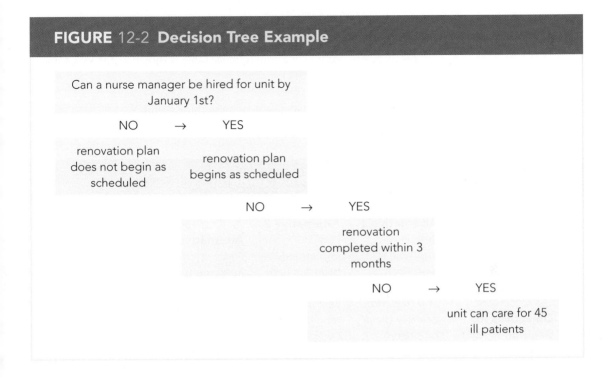

FIGURE 12-2 **Decision Tree Example**

Can a nurse manager be hired for unit by January 1st?

NO   →   YES

renovation plan does not begin as scheduled   renovation plan begins as scheduled

NO   →   YES

renovation completed within 3 months

NO   →   YES

unit can care for 45 ill patients

‹ Decision grid: This allows decision-makers to visually examine alternatives and compare them using a set of criteria. The same criteria will be used to assess each alternative. Criteria could include, for example, financial resources required, personnel commitment needed, and the public relations commitment needed to "sell" the decision to the media.

‹ Payoff tables: These allow cost, profit, and volume to be considered along with how they influence each other. They are used with historical data as well as probabilities. For example, if the decision in question is whether or not to change vendors of the hospital's supply of alcohol prep pads, the decision-makers will need information such as how many prep pads the hospital used each month for the past 6 months, the cost of one box of pads, the cost of the hospital's supply of pads for 6 months, as well as how many, if any, had to discarded as defective. These numbers allow the decision-maker to predict how many the hospital will likely use for the next 6 months.

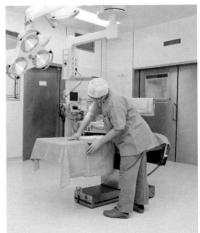

< Consequence tables: This lists the objectives for a decision down one side of a table and then rates how each potential alternative could fulfill each objective. An example of a consequence table is shown as **Table 12-3** (Marquis & Huston, 2012).

Table 12-4 shows these tools that aid in the decision-making process.

TABLE 12-3 Example of Consequence Table

Objectives for Decision (should facility implement a wound care program?)	Alternative 1 (Yes, implement a program immediately and have the primary focus on prevention of hospital acquired pressure ulcers)	Alternative 2 (Yes, but don't implement the program until January of next year after the renovation is completed and more fiscal resources are available)	Alternative 3 (Yes, implement a program immediately and have the primary focus on prevention of diabetic foot ulcers)	Alternative 4 (No, such a program is not needed at this time)
Reduce number of patients developing hospital-acquired pressure ulcers				
Reduce number of patients experiencing long-term complications from pressure ulcers				
Reduce number of diabetic patients experiencing skin care issues				
Comply with all Joint Commission requirements regarding skin care				

Source: Marquis & Huston, 2012.

TABLE 12-4 Tools to Aid in the Decision-Making Process

Tool	Description	Effect on Decision-Making
Trial and error	The RN selects a likely solution and tries it.	This is not a good choice for a nurse manager to utilize consistently, since it gives the impression of the manager being ineffective and not understanding how evidence translates into practice. Frequent use of trial-and-error expends a great deal of unit resources, and it can be very expensive making corrections after realizing that the wrong solution was chosen yet again.
Pilot projects	The RN does a trial run with a solution using a small number of participants.	This can be a wise choice if the nurse manager is reasonably certain that this will be the chosen alternative or some variation of it. Because the number of participants is small, few resources (money, personnel, time, effort) are expended and thus even if the choice does not provide to be effective, the loss is small. Problems are detected early and either can be rectified or may be cause to discard the alternative in favor of one with fewer difficulties.
Creativity techniques	These can include brainstorming, the Delphi process and nominal group techniques. These work particularly well with a complicated problem that has no clear-cut solution. The goal in this case is to generate potential solution without the encumbrance of possible bias.	These should be used with any problem that does not have a clear-cut solution. Since participants must be able to think "outside the box," the techniques will not work well with participants who exhibit very concrete thinking.
Decision tree	This is a model that allows the nurse to visualize the alternatives available as well as the various outcomes that can occur. Usually a question will be asked with various options that could result branching below.	This will work best with participants who can think creatively and thus generate multiple alternatively and various outcomes. Participants also must be able to demonstrate long-range thinking and thus anticipate possible outcomes.

Tool	Description	Effect on Decision-Making
Scenario planning	This works well with situations that change frequently. It asks the question "What if?," and therefore allows for the development of a wide variety of possible outcomes.	This is a strategy that works well with groups of creative participants who must be able to generate multiple possible outcomes. Participants must be able to "brainstorm" areas for further development of the facility as well as areas that would be overly risky to venture into.
Worst-case scenario	This is particularly useful when considering decisions that involve risk. This allows alternatives with their potential consequences to be ranked as "most desirable" and "least desirable."	This will be most successful with participants who have enough of an understanding of how the unit works to be able to consider how a deteriorating situation could truly progress to the point of disaster. Participants must also be able to consider the long-term effects of implementing a specific decision versus a different choice.
Decision grid	This allows decision-makers to visually examine alternatives and compare them using a set of criteria. The same criteria will be used to assess each alternative.	Participants must be capable to applying the same criteria to all alternatives, therefore, training may be required in areas such as financial resources, allocation of personnel, and educational requirements needed to achieve objectives.
Payoff tables	These allow cost, profit, and volume to be considered along with how they will influence each other.	In order to utilize these to their maximum potential, participants should have a working knowledge of the historical data associated with the unit in question. If participants do not have an understanding of the unit's cost, profit, and volume and how these are generated, there will be difficulty forecasting future numbers in these areas.
Consequence tables	This lists the objectives for a decision down one side of a table and then rates how each potential alternative could fulfill each objective.	This will work most effectively with participants who can think creatively and thus generate multiple alternatives. Also, creativity will be required to determine how each alternative could meet required objectives.

Source: Marquis & Huston, 2012.

Summary of Key Points in Chapter

The chapter discussed the basic steps in the decision-making process. The difference between clinical judgment, critical thinking, decision-making, and problem solving was also delineated. Factors that could potentially serve as obstacles to the decision-making process, including those unique to the individual, were described. Various types of group decision-making were discussed. Finally, various types of tools that could assist in the decision-making process were described.

Conclusion

The ability to make decisions that incorporate critical thinking, clinical judgment, and problem solving may well be symbolic of the pinnacle of success for a nurse manager or leader. A nurse that can successfully make decisions is capable of communicating effectively, incorporating change appropriately, engaging in health promotion, being sensitive to various cultures, and functioning in multiple roles in health care.

Critical Thinking Questions

1. Compare and contrast problem solving and decision-making.
2. Compare and contrast critical thinking and clinical judgment.
3. Consider your current work situation. Can you think of a time when a nurse leader had a difficult time making a decision? Do you believe any of the "obstacle" criteria played a part in the difficulty?
4. Think of a decision you recently made. Which aspects of you as an individual were involved in making the decision? Consider the alternatives you evaluated when making the decision. What factors were involved in your final decision?
5. Consider your individual thinking style. Are you left or right brain dominant? Explain your answer.

Scenarios

1. You are caring for Mrs. Sanchez, a 21-year-old patient who came into the emergency department this evening in labor with her sixth baby.

She speaks only Spanish and is accompanied by her mother and her husband. Her mother also speaks only Spanish. Her husband speaks some very basic English. The obstetrician on call wants to take the patient to surgery for a cesarean section because her blood pressure is 180/110 and is continuing to climb. How can you convey this to the patient and her family so informed consent can be given? Use the steps of the decision-making process to make a decision:

2. You are caring for Mr. McQueen, a patient who had surgery yesterday for a ruptured appendix. His recovery has been progressing without incident until a few moments ago, when he began to complain of feeling faint. His blood pressure is 90/50, and his pulse is 116. He is pale and sweating. He tells you he just urinated in his urinal, and you note that he produced 500 ml of bright red urine. You go to notify the charge nurse, who tells you, "I guess you're in charge now—I just quit!" What should you do? Use the steps of the decision-making process to make a decision.

3. You are a unit manager, and the hospital administrator has approached you about changing the staff from working 8-hour shifts to working 12-hours shifts. However, the change will not be implemented unless the staff is in agreement about the change. Describe the process of making such a decision using the

   a. Nominal group technique

   b. Delphi group technique

   c. Consensus-building technique

4. You are the director of critical care services for a 400-bed metropolitan hospital. You are the chairperson of a committee that is struggling with deciding if the facility needs to move to an electronic charting system and, if so, which system should be used. Use the following tools to help the committee make a decision:

   a. Trial and error

   b. Pilot projects

   c. Creativity techniques

   d. Decision tree

   e. Scenario planning

   f. Worst-case scenario

   g. Decision grid

   h. Payoff tables

   i. Consequence tables

NCLEX® Questions

Using the information you obtained from studying this chapter, go online to complete the following NCLEX®-format review questions. Visit http://go.jblearning.com/terryLPN using the access code in the front cover of your book. This interactive resource allows you to answer each question and instantly review your results. Practice until you can answer at least 75% successfully, and then try to improve your score with each successive attempt.

Match the descriptor with the appropriate strategy to aid in decision-making. Strategies can be used more than once.

1. _____ this is a group strategy that works well with situations that change frequently

2. _____ the RN chooses a solution that seems to be a likely choice and tries it

3. _____ the goal for the strategy is to generate potential solutions without the burden of possible bias

4. _____ this strategy lists the objectives for a decision down one side of a table and then rates how each potential alternative could fulfill each objective

5. _____ model that allows the nurse to visualize the alternatives available as well as various outcomes that can occur

6. _____ the nurse manager who uses this as a decision-making method is perceived as ineffective and having a poor grasp of evidence-based practice

7. _____ this strategy asks the question "what if?" and therefore allows for the development of a wide variety of possible outcomes

8. _____ asks a question with various options that could result in branching

9. _____ strategy that is especially useful when considering decisions that involve risk

10. _____ the RN tries a solution with a small number of participants as a limited trial

11. _____ allows the technique to progress to the point of having everything that possibly could go wrong culminate in disaster simultaneously

12. _____ this strategy allows the nurse to try a solution on a limited basis so that major problems can be detected early, minimizing risk

13. _____ allows a facility to foreshadow the possible long-range effects of implementing a certain decision

14. _____ allows decision-makers to visually examine alternatives and compare them using a set of criteria

15. _____ uses criteria such as financial resources and personnel commitment to assess each alternative

16. _____ allow cost, profit, and volume to be considered along with how they influence each other

17. _____ can include brainstorming, the Delphi process, and nominal group techniques

18. _____ can be used to allow the decision-maker to predict how many supplies a hospital would use over a specific period of time

19. _____ uses cost, profit, volume, historical data and probabilities

20. _____ this strategy works particularly well with a complicated problem without a clear-cut solution

Strategies:

a. trial and error
b. pilot projects
c. creativity techniques
d. scenario planning
e. decision tree
f. worst-case scenario
g. payoff tables
h. consequence tables
i. decision grid

For more information on the topics in this chapter and others, please see Appendix on p. 299 for a list of web links to additional resources.

References

Gillespie, M. (2010). Using the situated clinical decision-making framework to guide analysis of nurses' clinical decision-making. *Nurse Education in Practice, 10,* 333–340.

Huber, D. (2010). *Leadership and nursing care management* (4th ed.). Maryland Heights, MO: Elsevier.

Kelly, P. (2010). *Essentials of nursing leadership and management* (2nd ed.). Clifton Park, NY: Delmar.

Marquis, B. L., & Huston, C. J. (2012). *Leadership roles and management functions in nursing* (7th ed.). Philadelphia, PA: Lippincott Williams & Wilkins.

Missri, E. (2008). Gender Differences in Decision Making Processes: A Computerized Experiment. Retrieved from http://portal.idc.ac.il/en/schools /Government/politicalpsychology/Documents/gender_differences_in _decision_making_processes.pdf

For a full suite of assignments and additional learning activities, use the access code located in the front of your book to visit this exclusive website: http://go. jblearning.com/terryLPN. If you do not have an access code, you can obtain one at the site.

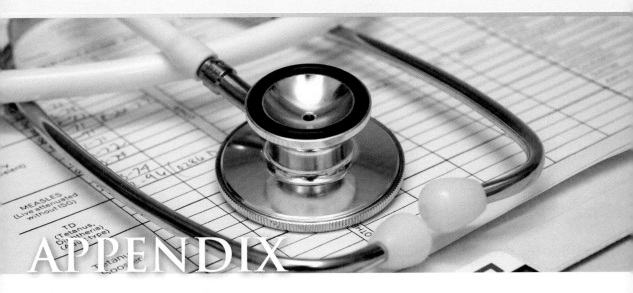

APPENDIX

Web Links to Topics

Magnet Hospitals

1. www.nursecredentialing.org/Magnet.aspx
2. www.nursecredentialing.org/Magnet
   /ResourceCenters/MagnetResearch/DEO-
   FAQ.aspx

NCLEX Preparation

1. https://www.ncsbn.org/nclex.htm
2. https://www.ncsbn.org/2010_NCLEX_RN
   _Detailed_Test_Plan_Candidate

Communication in Nursing

1. www.patientprovidercommunication.org
   /index.cfm/article_9.htm
2. www.rwjf.org/pr/product.jsp?id=30312

Professional Associations

1. www.nursingworld.org/
2. www.nursingsociety.org/
3. www.aanp.org/AANPCMS2
4. www.wocn.org

5. www.ons.org
6. www.nln.org
7. www.nbna.org
8. www.aamn.org

Lobbying in Nursing

1. www.maction.org/site/PageServer?
   pagename=nstat_take_action_activist_tool-
   kit&ct=1&ct=1
2. www.nursingworld.org/MainMenu
   Categories/ANAPoliticalPower.aspx

Models of Nursing Care

1. www.loyolamedicine.org/Medical_Services
   /Features/Nursing_Care_Model.cfm
2. www.nicheprogram.org
3. www.hartfordign.org/programs/niche
   /index.html
4. www.currentnursing.com/nursing_theory
   /models_of_nursing_care_delivery.html

Safety in Nursing Practice

1. https://www.nursingquality.org
2. www.jointcommission.org
3. www.ahrq.gov

Nursing Process

1. www.netplaces.com/new-nurse/what-you-learned-in-school/the-nursing-process.htm
2. www.sabacare.com/Frameweek/Nursing Process.html

Change Process in Nursing

1. www.nursing-informatics.com/changemant.html
2. www.nursing-informatics.com/kwantlen/wwwsites3.html

Health Promotion in Nursing

1. www.who.int/topics/health_promotion/en/
2. www.cdc.gov/healthyliving/

Legal and Ethical Aspects of Nursing

1. http://www.hhs.gov/ocr/hipaa/
2. http://www.nursingworld.org/
3. http://bioethics.od.nih.gov/
4. http://depts.washington.edu/bioethx/topics/index.html

Cultural Considerations in Nursing

1. www.transculturalcare.net/ethics.htm
2. http://www.culturediversity.org/
3. http://erc.msh.org/
4. http://www.omhrc.gov/
5. http://www.hrsa.gov/culturalcompetence/

Evidence-Based Practice

1. www.libguides.hsl.washington.edu/ebp
2. www.asha.org/members/ebp/

3. www.hsl.unc.edu/Services/Tutorials/EBM/whatis.htm
4. www.ahrq.gov
5. www.evidence.anc.umn.edu/
6. http://www.ahrq.gov/clinic/epcix.htm

Decision-Making Process in Nursing

1. www.scu.edu/ethics/practicing/decision/
2. www.ethicsweb.ca/resources/decision-making/index.html

Roles of the Registered Nurse

1. www.leadingtoday.org/weleadinlearning/jrapr03.htm
2. www.discovernursing.com
3. www.explorehealthcareers.org/en/Career/148/Nurse_Researcher

Dosages and Solutions

1. www.mcalc.com/
2. www.dosagehelp.com/

Jean Watson

1. http://currentnursing.com/nursing_theory/Watson.html
2. http://www.watsoncaringscience.org/

Leadership Role of the RN

1. http://www.nurseleader.com/
2. http://www.reflectionsonnursingleadership.org/pages/vol35_3_sieg_nursingleaders.aspx

Novice to Expert

1. http://currentnursing.com/nursing_theory/Patricia_Benner_From_Novice_to_Expert.html
2. http://library.stritch.edu/research/subjects/health/nursingTheorists/benner.html

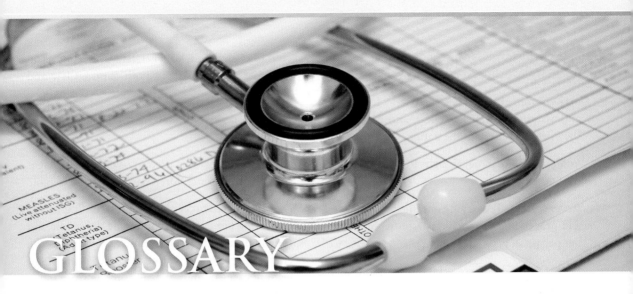

GLOSSARY

acculturation: Members of a minority group usually assume the beliefs, practices, and values of the dominant cultural group in the society so that a blending of the cultural group occurs. The person accepts both his or her own culture and the new one and therefore assumes aspects of both cultures.

ACE star model: Provides a framework within which to organize the various concepts included in evidence-based practice as they progress toward knowledge transformation.

action: In this stage of the transtheoretical model of change, the individual has made obvious changes in his or her lifestyle within the past 6 months. The goal at this point is to reach a standard that health professionals have agreed on as being adequate to sufficiently reduce the risk for disease. This stage is also crucial because of the monitoring to prevent relapse that must occur.

active listening: Occurs when the hearer recognizes and acknowledges the person sending the message is conveying an important transmission, whether the receiver agrees with it or not.

administrative law: Deals with protecting the rights of citizens.

advanced directives: Set of instructions to relay a person's wishes about health care if he or she were unable to make and verbalize a decision.

advanced practice nurses: Nurse practitioners, nurse midwives, or certified registered nurse anesthetists.

affective domain: Involves feelings, values, and attitudes.

alcohol/substance abuse by a nurse: Common reason for a nurse to sustain discipline against his or her license.

American Nurse Association Code of Ethics: Provides guidance to the nurse on various types of ethical issues.

Annie G. Fox: World War II–era nurse who became the first Army nurse to receive the Purple Heart.

assault: Threatening to touch another person, such as a patient, in a manner that is offensive to that person and without his or her permission.

assessment: Involves data collection on the various health issues being experienced by the patient.

assimilation: Individuals choose to learn about and assume the values, beliefs, and behaviors of the primary culture of the nation.

autonomy: The patient's right to make his or her own decisions.

battery: Actually carrying out the threat of assault and proceeding to touch a person without his or her permission.

beneficence: The nurse wants to do good for the patient and balances the potential benefit to the patient with the potential risk.

biomedical view: Proposes that illness is caused by germs, viruses, or some type of breakdown in the basic functioning of the body.

Bloom's taxonomy: Consists of domains of learning.

Brahmanism: System of religious beliefs, also known as Hinduism. Also provided teachings related to hygiene, the prevention of illness, medicine, and surgery.

case presentations: May be helpful in teaching the nursing student how to complete patient histories, develop nursing diagnoses, and interpret laboratory findings.

challenge: The individual believes that change is positive and thus is challenged by stressful situations and daily disruptions because they cause him or her to grow as a person and develop new coping strategies.

change agent: Leads staff in implementation of the change process.

channel of communication: Direction in which the message is routed to receivers.

civil law: How individuals relate to each other in daily life, and consists of both contract law and tort law.

Clara Barton: Founder of the American Red Cross.

Clark's rule: Formula used in calculating dosages of medication for children based on body weight.

clinical nurse leader: Way of responding to the increasing level of care required by the public and the changes in the healthcare environment. The clinical nurse leader is intended to be capable of leading in all settings of healthcare delivery but is not intended to be an administrative or management position.

clinical trials: Various testing phases for new drugs used in the treatment of cancer patients.

cognitive domain: Involves knowledge and intellectual skill.

Colonel Anna May Hays: Led Army nurses in Vietnam; promoted to Brigadier General in 1970. Colonel Hays became the first nurse in American military history to attain general officer rank.

Colonel Mildred Clark: Led Army nurses in Vietnam along with Colonel Anna May Hays.

commitment: The individual is immersed in the activities of life, believes what he does is both interesting and important, and actively engages in problem-solving to improve the work environment for all employees, not only himself.

communication: Exchange of information that can occur through speech, writing, signals, or behavior.

conceptual framework: Defines the patient, environment, health, and nursing, and this directs the way is which nursing care is delivered within the confines of the nursing process.

confidentiality: Pertains to the amount of information that can be disclosed about a patient without his consent.

consensus building: A type of group decision-making technique in which all group members may not be in complete agreement with all aspects of the decision that has been made but they are capable of being supportive of that decision.

constitutional law: A citizen's rights, privileges, and responsibilities provided through the Constitution of the United States, including those documented in the Bill of Rights.

contemplation: In this stage of the transtheoretical model of change, the individual has intentions of changing his or her behavior at some point in the next 6 months. He or she is equally aware of the advantages and disadvantages of changing the behavior. This awareness can promote ambivalence in the individual and can cause him or her to be labeled as a procrastinator.

contextual stimuli: All other stimuli present that contribute to the effect of the focal stimuli in Rogers' theory of nursing.

continuous change: Type of change that occurs on an incremental basis so it is always evolving toward the final intended outcome; the results of each incremental change are cumulative.

contract law: Regulates certain types of transactions between individuals and businesses as well as transactions between businesses.

control: The individual has a high degree of control because he believes that he can influence the level of stress that he is experiencing and thus can change the factors producing it.

criminal conviction of a nurse: Nurses can receive discipline from their state boards of nursing if they receive criminal convictions, are convicted of a felony, or are convicted of any type of crime involving gross immorality. This can include fraud, misrepresentation, embezzlement of funds, patient abuse, and murder.

criminal law: Actions of individuals that are intentionally directed to harm members of the public.

critical thinking: Ability to examine the evidence provided, use reasoning to analyze it, and then develop a judgment about the evidence.

cues to action: In the health belief model, anything that motivates the person to take action to begin incorporating health-promoting behaviors.

cultural awareness: Occurs when the nurse examines his or her own background to recognize the existence of biases, prejudices, and assumptions that are present about other people. An examination and exploration of the nurse's cultural and professional background that result in recognizing the nurse's biases, prejudices, and assumptions about people who are different.

cultural competence: Providing nursing care that is designed specifically for a patient, is inclusive of that patient's cultural norms and values, assists the person in making his or her own decisions regarding health care, and is sensitive to the patient's unique culture.

cultural desire: Nurse's motivation to become culturally aware, knowledgeable, and skillful; also encompasses the concept of caring.

cultural diversity: Variations that can be observed between cultures.

cultural encounter: Process used by the nurse to interact with a patient from a different cultural background; can cause the registered nurse to change his or her current beliefs about a cultural group and help the nurse avoid stereotyping the patient.

cultural knowledge: Acquired through the process of obtaining research-based information about different cultures and ethnic groups.

cultural skill: Ability to accurately perform a cultural assessment and collect relevant cultural data about the patient's current problem.

cultural universality: Similarities that exist in various cultures when they are subjected to scrutiny.

culturally congruent care: Nursing care that respects the patient's values and life patterns.

culture: Interwoven pattern of a person's behavior made up of language, thoughts, mode of communication, actions, customs, belief system, values, and institutions unique to his or her racial and ethnic makeup and chosen religious and social groups.

culture shock: Develops when a person emigrates from one culture to another and finds his or her belief system and values are not highly esteemed by the new culture.

deaconess: Prototype for the modern community health nurse after the third century A.D. during the Christian era.

Deborah: First nurse mentioned by name in recorded history. Her name was recorded in the 24th chapter of the book of Genesis as being the nurse of Rebekah.

decision-making: Choosing a certain course of action.

decisive decision-making: Does not require a large amount of available information to make a decision.

decoding: Occurs as the receiver interprets the message in an attempt to make it meaningful.

Delphi group technique: Uses questionnaires to obtain group members' opinions. The responses are summarized and then distributed to group members repeatedly until group consensus is achieved. Because this technique can be used with a large number of participants, it has the potential to generate a large number of ideas.

dependent nursing intervention: Requires supervision from another healthcare professional such as a physician to be implemented.

developmental change: Can be either planned or emergent and, like continuous change, develops incrementally over time.

diagonal communication: Channel of communication in which the registered nurse interacts with members of other departments in the facility.

diagnostic operation: In Orem's theory, establishes the nurse–patient relationship and determines the individual's ability to provide self-care.

discovery: Stage of the ACE star model when new knowledge is being produced by research methods used in original research studies.

doctor of nursing practice: Clinical doctorate for nurses that ideally puts them on the same level with other professions that require a practice doctorate, such as medicine and dentistry.

domain: Categories of learning as described in Bloom's taxonomy.

"do not resuscitate" orders: A written order that indicates whether a patient wants to be resuscitated in the event of a deteriorating physical condition.

Dorothea Dix: Developed a set of qualifications for nurses as part of her work as the superintendent of female nurses for the Union Army during the Civil War.

downward communication: The registered nurse sends the message to subordinates.

drop factor: Number of drops per milliliter of liquid; it is determined by the size of the drops.

due process: Discipline of the nurse's license cannot occur without following a previously established legal procedure.

durable power of attorney: Exists when a competent person names another person to make decisions about his or her health care if he or she is unable to do so. The document frequently gives specific instructions about feeding tubes, cardiopulmonary resuscitation, and being placed on ventilators; must be witnessed by two people.

early adopter: Consulted regarding information about changes that are occurring because of the high esteem with which he or she is held by colleagues; this person can be one of the greatest allies of the change agent.

early majority: Has a preference for what was done in the past but will accept the new status quo created by the change; this person is supportive of the actions of the change agent but may be reluctant to move the change process too quickly or to make more than incremental changes.

evaluation: State of the ACE star model when the effectiveness of the change in nursing practice should be evaluated by the patient population, the healthcare provider, and the overall healthcare system.

Edith Nourse Rogers: Congresswoman who introduced the Women's Auxiliary Army Corps bill into Congress in 1941.

Ednah Dow Cheney: Founded the New England hospital for women and children along with Marie Zakrzewska.

Edwin Smith Surgical Papyrus: Earliest known surgical prototype textbook that lists the proper surgical treatment for a variety of traumatic injuries.

emergency assessment: Used when time is of the essence due to the life-threatening nature of the patient's problem. It includes only essential data relevant to the patient's immediate issue.

emergent change: This is change that occurs spontaneously. It is unplanned and subsequently may be unable to be controlled; may not involve a change agent.

encoding: Sender translates his or her ideas into actual language.

encrypted: Process of coding sensitive information before it is put out onto the Internet to prevent it from being accessed by parties who should not view it.

energy field: The basic unit of both the living and nonliving entities in the universe in Rogers' theory of nursing.

episodic change: This type of change occurs because it was planned and is intended to occur on an occasional basis.

ethical dilemma: A conflict between two separate ethical duties owed to the patient, the patient's rights and the benefits that he or she could expect, a duty owed to the nurse and the duty owed to the patient, and professional ethical requirements and religious beliefs of the nurse.

ethnicity: Awareness of belonging to a specific group.

euthanasia: Deliberate ending of life in the interest of ending the suffering of the patient.

evaluating: Involves a judgment of the extent to which the change process is progressing toward the intended outcome.

evaluation: Stage when the registered nurse decides if the goals that he or she developed in collaboration with the patient were actually fulfilled.

evidence-based practice: Consistent use of research-based information in making decisions about patient care delivery.

evidence summary: Stage of the ACE star model when evidence from all research studies available is combined so the nurse researcher has the current scientific view of the topic.

exploitation phase: In Peplau's theory, phase of the nurse–patient relationship that uses professional resources to assist in designing problem-solving alternatives.

external climate: Exists for both the sender and the receiver and consists of the weather conditions, temperature, timing, and overall organizational climate of the facility in addition to the status of the person involved, level of power, and degree of authority wielded.

extrapersonal stressor: Occurs in the external environment outside of the client system but farther away from the system boundaries.

feedback: Generated by a continuous process of data gathering.

fidelity: Pertains to being loyal to commitments that have been made and accountability for responsibilities.

flexible decision-making: Uses a small amount of data in decision-making, produces multiple alternatives, and may result in a change in the final decision if additional information is revealed or available information is reinterpreted.

Florence Nightingale: Founder of nursing as a profession as a result of her training at the Deaconess Institute and her work with the wounded during the Crimean War.

flow rate: Rate at which intravenous fluids are given; it is measured in drops per minute.

focal stimuli: Those that immediately confront the patient in Rogers' theory of nursing.

focused assessment: Performed on each problem once they are identified. This type of assessment is important because it allows symptoms to be examined in greater detail, promotes the weighing of various etiologies to explain those symptoms, searches for contributing factors, and examines patient characteristics that would also help solve the presenting problem or at least clarify the issue.

Force-Field Model of Change: Lewin's change theory of how the process of change unfolds in an organization.

Fried's rule: Formula used to calculates dosages of medication for children under the age of 2.

futile care: Care that seems to have no benefit for the patient.

general adaptation syndrome: According to Hans Selye, the responses of every person to prolonged stress that can trigger the development of physiological illness.

grapevine: Most informal channel of communication. It moves rapidly and may involve several people simultaneously with no discernible systematic route. The message tends to be distorted as it moves throughout the organization's informal network.

hardiness: A set of beliefs held by the individual about him- or herself and the world. It is a valuable tool because it changes the way in which the individual views stress and it also makes available coping strategies to deal with the degree of stress being experienced; first defined by Kobasa.

health belief model: Proposes four primary perceptions that influence an individual's decision to take action to prevent illness: the person is potentially vulnerable to developing an illness, the effects of developing such an illness would be serious, there is a specific behavior that can prevent the development of the illness, and the benefits acquired by reducing the risk will be greater than the disadvantages connected with integrating the new behavior

Health Insurance Portability and Accountability Act: Legislation that first brought the need to ensure confidentiality of sensitive patient information to the public's attention.

health promotion: Uses education to provide people with the knowledge needed to maintain their own health.

health risk appraisal: Type of questionnaire that evaluates the patient's risk for development of disease based on his or her current demographics, lifestyle, and health-related practices.

Healthy People 2020: Contains goals and objectives for America's health promotion and disease prevention and has provided a critical design for public health priorities and interventions for the past 30 years. Developed in an attempt to address the gaps in care for vulnerable populations and ultimately decrease the existing health disparities.

Helen Fairchild: World War I–era nurse who became well known through her diary, published posthumously, that detailed daily life caring for military patients.

hierarchic decision-making: Uses a large amount of information in making the decision but will identify one solution or one alternative.

holistic view: Proposes that illness results from a person's life failing to be in harmony with nature.

honeymoon phase: First phase of reality shock for the new registered nurse as the role of registered nurse is initially assumed.

horizontal communication: Channel of communication used when the registered nurse sends a message to others in the organization who are on the same level as him- or herself.

implementation: Stage of the ACE star model in which evidence influences clinical decision-making and begins to change nursing practice. Effective implementation cannot occur without considering efficiency (is it efficient to use in terms of cost, personnel, and time?), currency (is it timely for the patient population under consideration?), and usefulness (is it something that will be readily used by both the client and the nurse?).

incongruent message: One in which what the sender is communicating verbally does not seem to match the nonverbal message that is being sent.

identification phase: In Peplau's theory, phase of the nurse–patient relationship that involves interdependent goal setting by the nurse and patient.

implementing: Usually occurs after the plan is established. However, an unexpected change may require immediate implementation and subsequently a rapid change in the plan.

independent nursing intervention: Does not require either supervision by or collaboration with another healthcare professional to implement.

informal change agent: Works closely with the formal change agent during the change process.

initial assessment: Occurs upon initial assessment of the patient.

innovator: Enjoys change but may not completely comprehend the degree of instability that can be created in the workplace environment by change; this person is completely supportive of the change agent's actions but may try to move the process too quickly in his or her enthusiasm.

integrative decision-making: Uses all available data in the decision-making process and identifies multiple alternatives that can be used in arriving at a final decision.

interdependent nursing intervention: Requires collaboration with another healthcare professional to implement.

internal climate: Values, feelings, personality or temperament, and stress levels under which the message is sent.

interpersonal stressor: Occurs in the external environment outside of the client system but close to the system boundaries.

intrapersonal stressor: Internal stressor that occurs within the boundaries of the client's system.

intuitive decision-making: Uses a trial-and-error approach to decision-making. This approach does not work well with a change agent because it relies on focusing on the general feeling that the person derives from the alternative presented and tends to ignore available information.

Iowa model: Method of understanding how research must be considered within the entire healthcare system to guide practice decisions.

I-SBAR-R technique: Standardized procedure used when communicating vital information to a colleague in a situation such as a transfer.

judgment: Most definitive conclusion the nurse can determine.

justice: This equates to providing fair and equal treatment to all patients and that benefits, risks, and costs are equally distributed so no one group or individual bears the burden exclusively.

Kate Cumming: Served as administrator of mobile field hospitals for the Army of Tennessee during the Civil War.

laggard: Would rather continue to practice traditional methods and openly acknowledges resistance to new ideas; this person demonstrates resistance to the actions of the change agent and may be passive-aggressive in response.

late majority: Open about his or her negative feelings about the change and agrees to accept it only after others have accepted and incorporated it; this person demonstrates resistance to the actions of the change agent and may be passive-aggressive in response.

left-brain-dominant thinkers: Typically excel at tasks that require use of language, logic, numbers, and anything that uses sequential ordering.

Linda Richards: First trained nurse in America.

listening: Method by which the receiver becomes aware of the message communicated by the sender.

living will: A document prepared by a competent person that gives instructions about the medical care that should be provided for that person if he or she becomes unable to make and verbalize decisions. The person can also specify the types of health care used at the end of his life, such as specifying that he or she does not want to receive tube feedings if unable to eat.

magico-religious view: Holds that health and illness are the result of supernatural intervention.

maintenance: Stage of the transtheoretical model of change in which the individual works to prevent relapse. The person has confidence the change in behavior will continue.

malpractice: Consists of a professional's wrongful conduct in carrying out his or her duties as a professional, leading to harm ensuing to another person entrusted to his or her care.

Marie Zakrzewska: Founded the New England Hospital for women and children along with Ednah Dow Chaney.

Mary Eliza Mahoney: First African American professional nurse.

message: Information the sender communicates to the receiver.

mode of communication: Means of communicating the message, such as nonverbal, verbal, telephone, or written.

model: Documentation of the interaction that occurs between concepts and the patterns that result from that interaction.

modeling: When the preceptor demonstrates clinical expertise while caring for patients as the nursing student observes what's occurring.

moral courage: Remedy for moral distress.

moral distress: The nurse knows the right decision to make in a specific circumstance but is prevented from making the right decision by constraints imposed by the facility.

Mosaic law: Followed by the ancient Israelites from 15th century B.C. until the 1st century A.D. Responsibility for the health of the public rested with the male-dominated priestly tribe. The people were taught to prevent disease through personal hygiene and specific times for work, rest, and sleep. Specific instructions were provided regarding treatment of women during pregnancy, childbirth, and menstruation; selecting food that met dietary requirements; recognizing communicable disease; and when to implement quarantine procedures.

moving stage: Focuses on clearly identifying the issue at hand, the development of goals and objectives, and the development and implementation of strategies to meet the goals. This stage includes the development and encouragement of new values, attitudes, and behavior toward the proposed change.

multistate licensure compact: Allows an agreement to be developed between specific states to enable nurses licensed in one state to practice in the other state members of the compact agreement without being required to apply for a new license.

negative feedback: Consists of information that is indicative of the existence of a problem and the need to make a correction to either continue the progress made in the change process or to refocus the process so it is congruent with the original intended outcome.

negligence: Consists of failing to provide the care that a reasonable professional would provide in a similar situation.

New England Hospital for Women and Children: Teaching hospital for female physicians and later nurses run by an all-female staff that offered an education comparable with that received by male physicians.

nominal group technique: A type of group decision-making in which group members first write out their ideas about the issue in question and then present those ideas to the other group members along with the potential benefits and drawbacks.

nonmaleficence: Avoiding doing harm to the patient.

nontransactional conversation: Conversation that is not intended to have a specific purpose.

nonverbal communication: Mode of communication.

nurse advocate: Acts to protect patients from being abused and having their rights violated.

Nurse Practice Act: Gives each state's board of nursing the authority to define how nursing will be practiced in that locale, the educational preparation required to practice as either a licensed practical/vocational nurse or registered nurse in that state, and how professional nurses will be disciplined if they do not adhere to the rules governing nursing practice.

nursing diagnosis: Both measurable and realistic and used to direct the nursing process as it is individualized for the patient. A list of accepted nursing diagnoses was developed by the North American Nursing Diagnosis Association.

nursing goal: Determines the choice of nursing interventions to assist the patient in resolution of the problem and also indicates the amount of progress made toward resolution.

nursing process: Process through which assessment data are collected about a patient, nursing diagnoses are developed, goals and outcome criteria are created for each diagnosis, nursing interventions are selected for each diagnosis, and fulfillment of each goal is evaluated, thus creating a nursing plan of care for the patient.

nursing theory: Group of interrelated concepts and definitions that together describe a certain view of nursing.

objective data: Information about a patient that can be obtained through observation.

observation: Allows the student to watch as the preceptor interacts with patients, problem solves using critical thinking and nursing judgment, and moves through the nursing process.

ongoing assessment: Occurs throughout a patient's healthcare experience.

organizing: Involves making decisions using resources in the form of time, personnel, communication, or raw materials.

orientation phase: In Peplau's theory, problem-defining phase that starts when the client meets the nurse for the first time, with both being strangers.

outcome criteria: Specify the terms under which the goal will be met.

papyrus: Thick paper-like material.

patient cue: Either a specific response from the patient or the absence of a response that is appropriate for the specific patient situation.

Patient Self-Determination Act: Legislation that requires patients be given the opportunity to complete an advance directive if so desired.

Paula of Actin: Wealthy and learned Christian widow believed to be the first to train nurses systematically and to teach nursing as an art rather than as merely a service to the poor.

participative or consensus decision-making: This consists of actively attempting to involve others in the decision-making process, even if the decision is such that one individual must make the final decision. This style works well with a change agent monitoring the change process.

Pender's model of health promotion: Proposes that health is a dynamic state, ever in transition, and thus health promotion should strive to constantly increase the patient's well-being toward a higher level.

perceived barriers: In the health belief model, refer to the person's belief that although a new action may reduce likelihood of contracting a specific disease process, implementing the action may prove to be costly, whether in terms of actual funds, discomfort, or convenience.

perceived benefit: In the health belief model, the belief that there are advantages to use of the methods proposed for reducing the possibility of contracting the disease or reducing the seriousness of the illness resulting from the disease process.

perceived susceptibility: In the health belief model, the belief that one is potentially vulnerable to developing an illness.

perceived threat: In the health belief model, this consists of the patient's perceived susceptibility to illness combined with perceived severity of the potential illness.

planned change: This involves logical action that is based on deliberate reasoning; usually includes a formal change agent who is well versed in the change process.

planning: In this phase of the nursing process, the registered nurse prioritizes the diagnoses based on the immediate needs of the patient, such as airway, breathing, and circulation. Consists of looking ahead to decide on the most effective way to achieve a preset goal.

preceptor: Considered to be an experienced registered nurse who has proven his or her competence in nursing through performance in the work setting.

precontemplation: In this stage of the transtheoretical model of change, the individual does not intend to take action toward making a change in behavior for at least 6 months. The person may have already unsuccessfully attempted to change or may simply lack information about the consequences of his or her behavior and the subsequent need to change. At this stage the person does not want to discuss his or her behavior or consider the high-risk nature of choices being made. These people are frequently perceived as unmotivated or resistant to the idea of a change in behavior.

preparation: This stage in the transtheoretical model of change in which the individual intends to take action within the next month. The person usually has some type of plan of action and functions well in an active form of behavioral change

such as a weight loss program that relies heavily on exercise.

prescriptive operation: In Orem's theory, used in the planning stage when the nurse confirms with the patient that the baseline assessment is accurate and a plan of care is developed.

primary prevention: Focuses on behaviors that maintain wellness and prevent the development of illness. These interventions can include exercise classes, water safety classes, seminars on women's health, and heart-healthy meal planning.

privacy: Pertains to limiting the amount of information to disclose about oneself.

problem solving: Analyzing a specific situation.

process: Series of actions, proposed changes, or functions that are implemented to bring about a specific result.

proportion: An equation with a ratio on each side of the equal sign.

propositions: Statements used to explain relationships between the concepts used in a certain theory.

psychomotor domain: Involves physical movement, and thus learning in this category can be assessed according to distance, time, and speed.

public law: Includes constitutional law, criminal law, and administrative law.

ratio: Basically, a relationship of two numbers that exists in terms of size, amount, or quantity.

reality shock: Occurs when the new employee moves from the clearly defined role of the student into the more nebulous role of the registered nurse.

receiver: Interprets the meaning of the message based partially on the mode of communication used.

recovery phase: Phase of reality shock in which the new registered nurse shows evidence of making a smooth transition into his or her new role when he or she can evaluate the work environment objectively and predict how staff members usually will act in certain situations.

refreezing stage: Occurs when the change has become part of the work environment. The goal for this stage is to prevent a return to the past behavior patterns that resisted the change from occurring.

regulatory operation: In Orem's theory, used when the nurse designs and generates a system for nursing care for the patient that can range from completely compensatory, providing the highest level of care for the patient with little if any ability to provide self-care, to only supportive or educational, providing assistance to the individual who has the ability to provide self-care but needs additional knowledge.

rejector: Chooses to actively oppose change and may even sabotage the process being made toward a positive outcome; this person presents a challenge to the change agent because of his or her open resistance. The change agent may require the collaboration of other nurse leaders if this individual becomes particularly aggressive.

residual stimuli: In Rogers' theory of nursing, environmental factors that have not been determined in a specific situation.

resolution phase: In Peplau's theory, phase of the nurse–patient relationship in which the professional relationship with the nurse is terminated once the patient's needs have been met through collaboration between the nurse and the patient.

right-brain-dominant thinkers: Excel at tasks that require nonverbal ideas as well as those that pull concepts together into a whole structure.

role conflict: The stress that develops when the expectations of two different areas of authority over a nurse are not congruent.

Sally Louisa Tompkins: Founded Robertson Hospital in Richmond, Virginia during the Civil War and subsidized it primarily with her own funds.

scenario planning: Can be utilized as part of the decision making process.

secondary prevention: Focuses on diagnosing disease processes early, recognizing the existence of symptoms, and initiating treatment as rapidly as possible to avoid the development of complications.

self-efficacy: In the health belief model, the belief that the person believes that he or she is capable of implementing a new health-promoting behavior.

sender: Initiates the message that is sent to the receiver.

shock and rejection phase: Phase of reality shock that develops as the new registered nurse begins to recognize a conflict existing between what he or she was taught in the nursing program and what is actually occurring in the healthcare facility in daily practice.

socialized: The new member learns how to function as a member of a cultural group.

sterotyping: The nurse develops a distorted view of a particular group of people.

subjective data: Information about a patient that can only be gathered by interview.

systematic decision-making: Uses a structured approach to making decisions and a logical approach to forming the final decision.

taxonomy: System used to classify nursing diagnoses. The classification system yields 13 domains, which are then subdivided into classes and, ultimately, into diagnoses.

team decision-making: Focuses on bringing together collaborators' multiple ideas and experiences to produce a result that is much more extensive than the individual pieces of information that generated the decision. This can be a very effective style of decision-making when there is need for additional ideas or alternatives.

tertiary prevention: Focuses on rehabilitation after the development of a disease with the intent of preventing disability.

Theodor Fliedner: Revived the order of Deaconesses as prototype nurses and founded a hospital and training center at Kaiserswerth, Germany in 1836.

theoretical proposition: In Pender's model of health promotion, statements that act as a foundation for research to be performed on health behaviors.

theory of nursing systems: An attempt to explain the nature of relationships that must be both developed and maintained for nursing to be implemented.

theory of goal attainment: Nursing is a process by which the nurse and the client interact to develop a perception of each other and the client's situation and, as a result, develop goals for the client and collaborate on a means to achieve those goals.

theory of self-care: Describes why the individual will choose to care for him- or herself and how he or she will implement that care.

theory of self-care deficit: Explains why individuals can be helped through nursing and also describes how such care can be beneficial.

theory of transcultural nursing: Culture is learned, passed from one generation to the next, and can be observed in a person's actions, words, behavioral rules, and symbols.

Thomas Fuller: 18th century English physician who developed a set of qualifications for nurses.

tort: Negligent or intentional wrong not connected with a contract that injures a person and for which the injured party may opt to sue the responsible person for damages.

translation: Stage of the ACE star model in which clinical recommendations are generated that are both valid and reliable and are the result of evidence summaries combined with clinical expertise. By the conclusion of this stage, knowledge now reflects best practice and is based on evidence, consensus, and the endorsement of experts in the field. In this stage a healthcare agency may choose to adopt practice guidelines specific to a certain patient population.

transformational change: Like transitional change, considered to be radical in nature, but like emergent change, may be uncontrolled during the period of time that it takes the change to develop. The new changed condition will develop after the deterioration of the old condition.

transitional change: Occurs in planned episodes and usually is radical in nature.

transtheoretical model of change: Focuses on the decision-making ability of the individual to make an intentional change in his or her behavior. It proposes that a change in behavior is a process that occurs over time.

trial and error: The registered nurse selects a solution that seems to be a likely choice and tries it.

unethical/unprofessional practice by a nurse: This area can include breach of patient confidentiality, engaging in sexual relations with patients, initiating sexual harassment of patients or staff members, and discriminating against a patient based on his or her ethnicity, religion, or other significant characteristics; common reason for a state's board of nursing to bring discipline against a nurse's license.

unfreezing stage: Focuses on developing awareness of the problem and recognizing and decreasing the forces that are trying to maintain the status quo.

unilateral decision-making: This consists of one person making a decision with limited input from other colleagues. This style usually does not work well in a large healthcare organization with multiple stakeholders who are all affected by any type of decision as well as the smallest incremental change.

unitary human being: In Rogers' theory, an integration of the human being and his or her environment.

unprofessional conduct by a nurse: Conduct that is likely to deceive or harm the public, such as when a person uses false documentation to obtain a nursing license; common reason for a state's board of nursing to bring discipline against a nurse's license.

unsafe practice by a nurse: Negligence occurs in care delivery, resulting in delivery of incompetent care. State boards of nursing will initiate disciplinary actions against nurses for malpractice as well as negligence in practice.

upward communication: The registered nurse sends the message to a higher level.

Valentine Seaman: Developed the first formal instructional program for nurses in America.

veracity: Pertains to avoiding misleading patients.

verbal communication: Mode of communication.

vision: Basic concept that provides direction to implementation of the change.

Vivien Bullwinkel: Survived a massacre of Australian nurses in World War II Indonesia by Japanese forces.

vulnerable populations: Groups of individuals who are likely to develop health problems and experience poor outcomes in response to nursing interventions and medical treatment as a result of diminished access to medical care, various types of stressors, and engaging in types of high-risk behavior.

whistle-blower: Nurse who brings the wrong-doing in an organization to the attention of the public.

widow: Prototype for the modern community health nurse after the third century A.D. during the Christian era.

workplace advocate: Nurse manager ensures the work environment is safe for employees to work in and also supportive of their growth both personally and professionally.

Young's rule: Formula used to calculate dosages of medication for children aged 2 to 12.

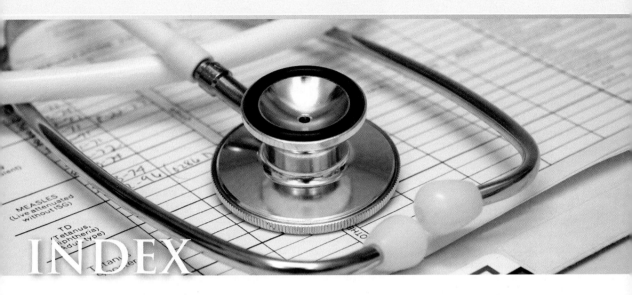

INDEX

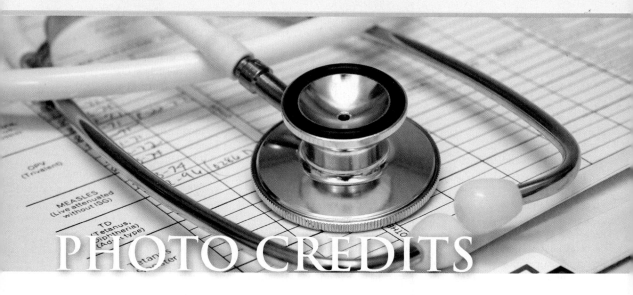

PHOTO CREDITS

CHAPTER 1

Page 6 © National Library of Medicine; page 7 © National Library of Medicine; page 12 © National Library of Medicine; page 14 © Ablestock.com/Thinkstock; page 16 © NorthGeorgiaMedia/ShutterStock, Inc.; page 16 © Photos.com; page 17 © Andy Dean Photography/ShutterStock, Inc.

CHAPTER 2

Page 30 © Yuri Arcurs/ShutterStock, Inc.; page 31 © Photos.com; page 37 © Ablestock.com/Thinkstock; page 42 © wavebreakmedia ltd/ShutterStock, Inc.; page 44 © Norma Pogson/ShutterStock, Inc.; page 45 © Yuri Arcurs/ShutterStock, Inc.

CHAPTER 3

Page 58 © Monkey Business Images/ShutterStock, Inc.; page 68 © Lisa F. Young/ShutterStock, Inc.; page 72 © Monkey Business Images/ShutterStock, Inc.; page 75 © Lisa S./ShutterStock, Inc.

CHAPTER 4

Page 87 © George Doyle/Stockbyte/Thinkstock; page 89 © iodrakon/ShutterStock, Inc.; page 92 © forestpath/ShutterStock, Inc.; page 98 © Alexander Raths/ShutterStock, Inc.; page 102 © Monkey Business Images/ShutterStock, Inc.

CHAPTER 5

Page 120 © George Doyle/Stockbyte/Thinkstock; page 124 © Thinkstock Images/Comstock/Thinkstock; page 126 © Blaj Gabriel/ShutterStock, Inc.; page 129 © Ramon grosso dolarea/ShutterStock, Inc.

CHAPTER 6

Page 145 © Phase4Photography/ShutterStock, Inc.; page 151 © Rmarmion/Dreamstime.com; page 155 © Comstock/Thinkstock.

CHAPTER 7

Page 170 © Kacso Sandor/ShutterStock, Inc.; page 171 © Dewayne Flowers/ShutterStock, Inc.; page 173 © Diego Cervo/ShutterStock, Inc.; page 176 © jordache/ShutterStock, Inc.; page 177 © Alexander Raths/ShutterStock, Inc.

CHAPTER 8

Page 98 © iStockphoto/Thinkstock; Page 199 © Vadym Drobot/ShutterStock, Inc.; page 212 © Rob Marmio/ShutterStock, Inc.

CHAPTER 9

Page 222 © Blaj Gabriel/ShutterStock, Inc.; page 224 © Joseph Dilag/ShutterStock, Inc.; page 225 © Blaj Gabriel/ShutterStock, Inc.; page 227 © Lisa F. Young/ShutterStock, Inc.

Chapter 10

Page 238 © Stockbyte/Thinkstock; page 239 © Rob Marmion/ShutterStock, Inc.; page 240 © Monkey Business Images/ShutterStock, Inc.; page 241 © takayuki/ShutterStock, Inc.; page 243 © Rido/ShutterStock, Inc.

Chapter 11

Page 260 © wavebreakmedia lt/ShutterStock, Inc.; page 261 © Mikhail Tchkheidze/ShutterStock, Inc.; page 262 © Photos.com; page 271 © Sportstock/ShutterStock, Inc.; page 271 © wavebreakmedia ltd/ShutterStock, Inc.

CHAPTER 12

Page 282 © coka/ShutterStock, Inc.; page 289 © spfotocz/ShutterStock, Inc.

Some images in this book feature models. These models do not necessarily endorse, represent, or participate in the activities represented in the images.